DEFENSE, SECURITY AND STRATEGIES

THE NATIONAL BIOSURVEILLANCE INTEGRATION CENTER

ROLES, CHALLENGES, AND STRATEGIC PLAN

DEFENSE, SECURITY AND STRATEGIES

Additional books in this series can be found on Nova's website under the Series tab.

Additional e-books in this series can be found on Nova's website under the eBooks tab.

DEFENSE, SECURITY AND STRATEGIES

THE NATIONAL BIOSURVEILLANCE INTEGRATION CENTER

ROLES, CHALLENGES, AND STRATEGIC PLAN

NATASHA JENNINGS
EDITOR

New York

Library of Congress Cataloging-in-Publication Data

ISBN: 978-1-63484-924-1

Published by Nova Science Publishers, Inc. † New York

CONTENTS

PREFACE

The National Biosurveillance Integration Center (NBIC) has activities that support its integration mission, but faces challenges that limit its ability to enhance the national biosurveillance capability. A biological event, such as a naturally occurring pandemic or a terrorist attack with a weapon of mass destruction, could have catastrophic consequences for the nation. This potential threat underscores the importance of a national biosurveillance capability—that is, the ability to detect biological events of national significance to provide early warning and information to guide public health and emergency response. The 9/11 Commission Act of 2007 addresses this capability, in part, by creating NBIC within the Department of Homeland Security (DHS); it was tasked with integrating information from human health, animal, plant, food, and environmental monitoring systems across the federal government, to improve the likelihood of identifying a biological event at an early stage. This book discusses the extent to which NBIC is implementing its roles as a biosurveillance integrator, and options for improving such integration.

In: The National Biosurveillance Integration ... ISBN: 978-1-63484-924-1
Editor: Natasha Jennings

Chapter 1

BIOSURVEILLANCE: CHALLENGES AND OPTIONS FOR THE NATIONAL BIOSURVEILLANCE INTEGRATION CENTER*

United States Government Accountability Office

WHY GAO DID THIS STUDY

A biological event, such as a naturally occurring pandemic or a terrorist attack with a weapon of mass destruction, could have catastrophic consequences for the nation. This potential threat underscores the importance of a national biosurveillance capability— that is, the ability to detect biological events of national significance to provide early warning and information to guide public health and emergency response. The 9/11 Commission Act of 2007 addresses this capability, in part, by creating NBIC within the Department of Homeland Security (DHS); it was tasked with integrating information from human health, animal, plant, food, and environmental monitoring systems across the federal government, to improve the likelihood of identifying a biological event at an earlier stage. In recent years, NBIC's budget has ranged from $10 million to $13 million annually.

* This is an edited, reformatted and augmented version of the United States Government Accountability Office publication, GAO-15-793, dated September 2015.

GAO was asked to evaluate NBIC. This report discusses the (1) extent to which NBIC is implementing its roles as a biosurveillance integrator, and (2) options for improving such integration. To conduct this work, GAO reviewed NBIC products and activities; conducted interviews and surveyed 19 federal partners, 11 of which have key roles in biosurveillance; interviewed NBIC officials; and analyzed the 9/11 Commission Act, *NBIC Strategic Plan*, and *National Strategy for Biosurveillance*.

WHAT GAO RECOMMENDS

GAO is not making recommendations. GAO provided this draft to DHS and its federal partners who provided technical comments which were incorporated, as applicable.

WHAT GAO FOUND

The National Biosurveillance Integration Center (NBIC) has activities that support its integration mission, but faces challenges that limit its ability to enhance the national biosurveillance capability. In the Implementing Recommendations of the 9/11 Commission Act of 2007 (9/11 Commission Act) and *NBIC Strategic Plan*, GAO identified three roles that NBIC must fulfill to meet its biosurveillance integration mission. The following describes actions and challenges in each role:

- **Analyzer:** NBIC is to use technology and subject matter expertise, including using analytical tools, to meaningfully connect disparate datasets and information for earlier warning and better situational awareness of biological events. GAO found that NBIC produces reports on biological events using open-source data, but faces challenges obtaining data and creating meaningful new information. For example, most of the federal partners with key roles in biosurveillance (8 of 11) stated that NBIC's products help their agencies identify biological events to little or no extent, generally because they already obtain such information directly from other federal partners more quickly. In addition, data that could help to identify and characterize a biological event may not exist or are not in a usable form. Further, few federal partners (5 of 19) reported that they share the data they do have with NBIC, citing legal and regulatory restrictions, among other reasons.

- **Coordinator:** NBIC is to bring together partners across the federal biosurveillance community to enhance understanding of biological events. NBIC has developed procedures and activities to coordinate with partners, such as daily and biweekly calls, but faces challenges related to the limited partner participation in the center's activities, lack of partner personnel detailed to NBIC, and competing structures for convening federal partners. For example, although NBIC would like to obtain liaisons from each of its federal partners, only 3 of 19 partners provided NBIC with dedicated liaisons.
- **Innovator:** NBIC is to facilitate the development of new tools to address gaps in biosurveillance integration. GAO found that NBIC has efforts underway to develop some tools, such as pilot projects examining the use of social media data to identify health trends, but faces challenges prioritizing developmental efforts. For example, partners noted limitations in NBIC's ability to address gaps, like limited resources and the difficulty in prioritizing the center's innovation efforts because its partners have diverse needs.

GAO identified various options that could address these challenges, ranging from strengthening the center's ability to implement its current roles to repealing NBIC's statute. GAO also identified potential benefits and limitations with each option. For example, one option would be to provide NBIC with additional authorities to obtain data to better develop meaningful information; however this may also require additional investments. Another option is to not pursue national biosurveillance integration through NBIC and to consider designating one of the other federal partners with key roles in biosurveillance as the federal integrator. The options identified are not exhaustive, and some could be implemented together or in part. GAO did not evaluate the financial implications of each option, but acknowledges some options may require additional investment or shifting of resources or priorities to result in significant long lasting change.

ABBREVIATIONS

9/11 Commission Act	Implementing Recommendations of the 9/11 Commission Act of 2007
AFHSC	Armed Forces Health Surveillance Center
APHIS	Animal and Plant Health Inspection Service
ASPR	Assistant Secretary for Preparedness and Response
BATR	Biological Assessment and Threat Response
CBP	Customs and Border Protection
CDC	Centers for Disease Control and Prevention
DHS	Department of Homeland Security
DOD	Department of Defense
DOE	Department of Energy
DOI	Department of the Interior
DOS	Department of State
DOT	Department of Transportation
EPA	Environmental Protection Agency
EVD	Ebola virus disease
FDA	Food and Drug Administration
FSIS	Food Safety Inspection Service
HHS	Health and Human Services
HPAI	highly pathogenic avian influenza
I&A	Office of Intelligence and Analysis
IT	information technology
NBIC	National Biosurveillance Integration Center
NBIS	National Biosurveillance Integration System
NCMI	National Center for Medical Intelligence
NOAA	National Oceanic and Atmospheric Administration
ODNI	Office of the Director of National Intelligence
PEDv	porcine epidemic diarrhea virus
S&T Roadmap	*National Biosurveillance Science and Technology Roadmap*
USDA	Department of Agriculture
USGS	U.S. Geological Survey
USPS	U.S. Postal Service
VA	Department of Veterans Affairs
WHO	World Health Organization

September 24, 2015

Congressional Requesters:

A biological event, such as a naturally occurring pandemic or a terrorist attack with a weapon of mass destruction, could have catastrophic consequences for the nation. Although Ebola did not cause many U.S. casualties, the outbreak in West Africa from 2013 through 2015 underscored the importance of developing and maintaining a national biosurveillance capability—that is, the ability to detect biological events of national significance with the aim of providing early warning and better information to guide public health and other types of emergency response. Further, because the data needed to detect an emerging infectious disease or bioterrorism threat may come from a variety of sources, the ability to share and analyze data from multiple sources may help officials better collaborate to analyze data and quickly recognize the nature of a disease event and its scope.

The Implementing Recommendations of the 9/11 Commission Act of 2007 (9/11 Commission Act) established the National Biosurveillance Integration Center (NBIC) within the Department of Homeland Security (DHS); it was specifically tasked with integrating and analyzing information from human health, animal, plant, food, and environmental monitoring systems across the federal government and supporting the interagency biosurveillance community.[1] In analyzing this act, as well as the August 2012 *NBIC Strategic Plan*, we identified three general roles that NBIC, as a federal-level biosurveillance integrator, must carry out to achieve the duties and outcomes described by NBIC's authorizing legislation: (1) Analyzer, (2) Coordinator, and (3) Innovator.[2]

- As an Analyzer, NBIC is to use technological tools and subject matter expertise to develop shared situational awareness by creating meaningful new insights from disparate datasets and information that could not be gleaned in isolation.[3]
- As a Coordinator, NBIC is to bring together multi-disciplinary partners across interagency organizations to enhance understanding of new or potential biological events, such as through the collaborative development of products and services.
- As an Innovator, NBIC is to facilitate the development of new tools, technology, and approaches to address gaps in biosurveillance integration.

In December 2009, we reported that NBIC was not fully equipped to carry out its mission because it lacked key resources—data and personnel— from its partner agencies, which may have been at least partially the result of collaboration challenges it faced.[4] For example, some partners reported that they did not trust NBIC to use their information and resources appropriately, while others were not convinced of the value that working with NBIC provided because NBIC's mission was not clearly articulated. In order to help NBIC enhance and sustain collaboration, including the provision of data, personnel, and other resources, we recommended that NBIC develop a strategy for addressing barriers to collaboration and develop accountability mechanisms to monitor these efforts. As previously noted, in August 2012, NBIC issued the *NBIC Strategic Plan*, which is intended to provide NBIC's strategic vision, clarify the center's mission and purpose, articulate the value that NBIC seeks to provide to its partners, and lay the groundwork for setting interagency roles, responsibilities, and procedures. Further, in November 2014, NBIC completed its first biannual NBIC Federal Stakeholder Survey, which NBIC uses to assess the usefulness of its products and activities and to determine what improvements should be made on the basis of those results. We believe these actions addressed the recommendations in our prior report.

You expressed interest in determining what progress NBIC has made in contributing to the national biosurveillance capability. This report's objectives are:

1. To what extent is NBIC implementing its roles as a biosurveillance integrator?
2. What are options for improving federal biosurveillance integration, and what are their benefits and limitations?

To determine the extent to which NBIC is implementing its role as a biosurveillance integrator, we conducted structured interviews with 19 federal departments and their component agencies across 13 of the 14 departments and agencies that compose the National Biosurveillance Integration System (NBIS)—the federal partners that NBIC is responsible for coordinating because they have missions and resources that can contribute to earlier detection and shared situational awareness for biological events of national significance. Although NBIC has interaction with other stakeholders, we selected these 19 federal agencies based on their biosurveillance roles and responsibilities and because they were federal departments or components within federal departments that have signed the NBIC Advisory Board charter—signifying their participation in the NBIS.[5] Prior to conducting our structured interviews, we provided a list of these agencies to NBIC and senior NBIC officials agreed that the agencies we identified represented the partners with which the center had the most interaction and collaboration.[6] We discussed with these NBIS partners the extent to which NBIC has enhanced the national biosurveillance capability by carrying out its national integrator roles and any challenges the center has faced in doing so, including the extent to which NBIC's products and activities enhance the agency's situational awareness of biological events. Within these agencies, we interviewed officials who serve on NBIC's Advisory Board or its Interagency Working Group, as well as other relevant officials that regularly interact with NBIC, review the center's products, or participate in the center's activities.[7] As part of this review, we did not interview or survey NBIC's nonfederal stakeholders, such as state, local, tribal, or territorial agencies.

We also conducted a Web-based survey of the 19 agencies to identify the federal agencies from which they obtain information that contributes to their agency's situational awareness of biological events, the methods through which they share information from NBIC, and the extent to which they participate in NBIC activities. We obtained a 100 percent response rate on this survey. In the survey, we asked each agency whether it obtains information from each of the other agencies in our population, as well as which types of information it obtains from them (perception-, comprehension-, or projection-related information). We performed a network analysis of these survey data, which is a quantitative and graphical technique for identifying the underlying patterns in a complex system of relationships among entities of interest.[8] Additional information on our survey methodology can be found in Appendix II.

Further, we reviewed NBIC products, such as its daily Monitoring List e-mail and Biosurveillance Event Reports, and observed some NBIC activities, such as its daily and bi-weekly calls. We reviewed key documents that guide NBIC's activities and products, such as the August 2012 *NBIC Strategic Plan*, the July 2012 *National Strategy for Biosurveillance*, and the White House's Office of Science and Technology Policy's June 2013 *National Biosurveillance Science and Technology Roadmap (S&T Roadmap)*.[9] We also reviewed other relevant documents, such as NBIC's Advisory Board's charter, standard operating procedures for the center's activities and protocols, memorandums of understanding and interagency agreements between NBIC and its federal partners, the results of NBIC's Federal Stakeholder Survey, and evaluations of NBIC's pilot projects. We also interviewed NBIC officials to obtain their opinions on the extent to which NBIC is implementing its roles as a biosurveillance integrator and enhancing the national biosurveillance capability.

To identify options for improving federal biosurveillance integration, as well as their benefits and limitations, we examined the 9/11 Commission Act to identify tasks and responsibilities that NBIC, as a federal-level biosurveillance integrator, is to carry out. We analyzed documents that identify potential gaps and needs in biosurveillance integration, including the *National Strategy for Biosurveillance* and the *S&T Roadmap*. We also obtained information from our structured interviews with NBIC's federal partners on their views about what else, if anything, the center could be doing to better enhance the national biosurveillance capability. Given the challenges described by NBIC's federal partners, we identified options for policy or structural changes. Although these options are not exhaustive, they represent a range of potential actions that could be taken to better fulfill the biosurveillance integration mission described in the 9/11 Commission Act.

We conducted this performance audit from July 2014 to September 2015 in accordance with generally accepted government auditing standards. Those standards require that we plan and perform the audit to obtain sufficient, appropriate evidence to provide a reasonable basis for our findings and conclusions based on our audit objectives. We believe that the evidence obtained provides a reasonable basis for our findings and conclusions based on our audit objectives.

BACKGROUND

Biosurveillance Integration

According to the July 2012 *National Strategy for Biosurveillance*, biosurveillance is the ongoing process of gathering, integrating, interpreting, and communicating essential information related to all- hazards threats or disease activity affecting human, animal, or plant health, for the purpose of (1) achieving early detection and warning, (2) contributing to overall situational awareness of the health aspects of the incident, and (3) enabling better decision making at all levels. As defined in the *NBIC Strategic Plan*, biosurveillance integration is combining biosurveillance information from different sources and domains (e.g., human, animal, and plant health; food and environmental safety and security; and homeland security) to provide partners and stakeholders with a synthesized view of the information, and what it could mean.[10] The goal is to create new meaning—that is, to provide insights that cannot be gleaned in isolation, leading to earlier warning of emerging events and shared situational awareness.

Example of a Biological Event Monitored by the National Biosurveillance Integration Center

Middle East respiratory syndrome coronavirus (MERS-CoV)

Since first recognized in September 2012 in Saudi Arabia, MERS-CoV has been detected in nearly 30 countries, including the United States. As of July 2015, there have been more than 1,300 confirmed cases and over 500 deaths, the vast majority of which have been in Saudi Arabia. Two cases have been detected in the United States from patients who had recently travelled to Saudi Arabia.

MERS-CoV is characterized as a potentially severe respiratory illness and symptoms may include fever, cough, shortness of breath, congestion of the nose and throat, and diarrhea. Camels are considered the likely source for human infections. As of June 2015, human-to-human transmission has been limited and the risk of infection to travelers visiting the Arabian Peninsula is considered to be low.

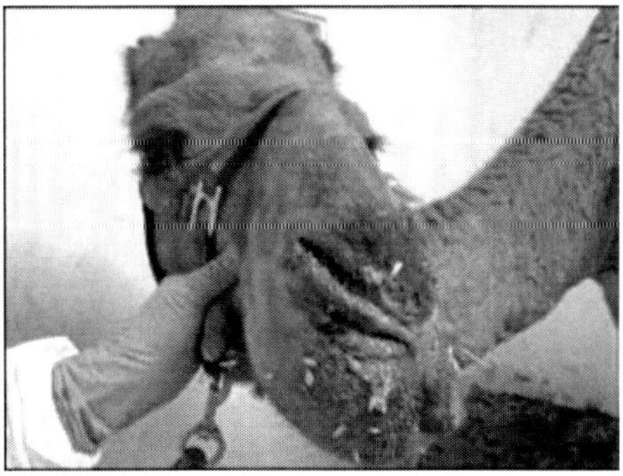

Source: National Biosurveillance Integration Center, Centers for Disease Control and Prevention (photo). | GAO 15-793

According to the *NBIC Strategic Plan*, biosurveillance, at a national level, is an important part of the process for achieving shared situational awareness of a biological event of national concern.[11] Situational awareness, which is composed of three related elements that are described in table 1, plays a critical role in enhancing common understanding and decision making. Emerging biological events often require that decisions be made based upon preliminary, incomplete, and often inconclusive information across multiple domains. Each department and agency in the biosurveillance community has a primary mission that is often focused on a single domain, yet decisions and actions must be made in a shared risk environment that considers all domains. According to the *NBIC Strategic Plan*, shared situational awareness across the biosurveillance community is achieved cooperatively by entities that integrate mission essential, overlapping portions of their individual situational awareness for a unified purpose, leading to a common picture or understanding of potential and ongoing biological events. Further, the plan notes that shared situational awareness of the broader biological domain may provide insights that cannot be gleaned in isolation, and thus enhance the likelihood of identifying an event earlier and with more certainty.

Table 1. Elements of Situational Awareness in the Biosurveillance Context

Element	Definition
Perception	The identification that a situation has occurred, such as the detection of a biological condition that differs from the norm. When such information is shared from one biosurveillance agency to another, it can help identify signals that a biological event with significance for an agency's mission might be occurring.
Comprehension	The understanding of the situation's meaning, such as the characterization of the nature and scope of the biological event. Shared information among biosurveillance agencies could help characterize and contextualize the nature and scope of an emerging biological event, which can help shape appropriate preparedness and response actions.
Projection	The determination of the event's likely course in the near future, such as how its nature and scope will evolve and the decision implications of that evolution. Such shared information among biosurveillance agencies could help understand how emerging and ongoing biological events are likely to progress in the near future, which can help subsequent decisions as to appropriate courses of action.

Source: GAO analysis of the Endsley Model of Situational Awareness and the *NBIC Strategic Plan*. | GAO-15-793

Note: For the purposes of this report, we use the definition of situational awareness that the *NBIC Strategic Plan* uses in the articulation of its mission. The definition has its basis in the work of Mica Endsley, a former Chief Scientist of the U.S. Air Force who has written extensively on situational awareness. For example, see Mica Endsley, "Toward a Theory of Situation Awareness in Dynamic Systems," Human Factors, vol. 37, no. 1 (1995), and Mica Endsley and Debra G. Jones, Designing for Situation Awareness: An Approach to User-Centered Design. 2nd ed., (Boca Raton, FL) CRC Press, 2011.

EXAMPLE OF A BIOLOGICAL EVENT MONITORED BY THE NATIONAL BIOSURVEILLANCE INTEGRATION CENTER

Highly pathogenic avian influenza (HPAI)

Since December 2014, the U.S. Department of Agriculture has confirmed 223 detections of HPAI in backyard and commercial poultry in 15 states. Over 48 million birds have been affected in the United States as of July 2015, making it the largest outbreak in the country's history. The export market for poultry products contributes billions of dollars to the U.S. economy annually. Import restrictions against U.S. poultry and poultry products by 52 countries and the European Union have resulted in decreases in some exports and local economic impacts, such as increases in egg prices and limited-scale layoffs.

HPAI is an infectious viral disease of wild birds and domestic poultry (e.g., chickens, turkeys, ducks, geese). Signs in birds include coughing, decreased egg production, and sudden death. Although some sub-types of HPAI can be transmitted to humans, no human infections in the United States have been recognized in association with the recent outbreak.

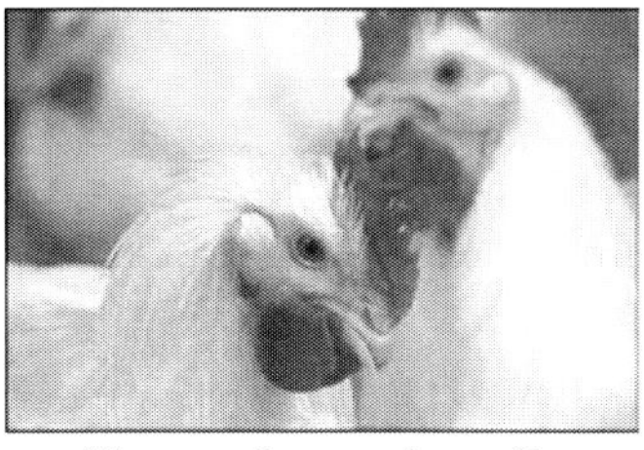

Source: National Biosurveillance Integration Center, U.S. Department of Agriculture (photo). | GAO 15-793

The importance of biosurveillance integration has also been described by key national planning documents. In July 2012, the White House issued the *National Strategy for Biosurveillance*, which describes the U.S. government's approach to strengthening biosurveillance. Although the strategy does not specifically identify roles for NBIC, it does emphasize the need for integration across disparate information sources, including data derived from intelligence, law enforcement, environmental, plant, animal, and other relevant areas. In June 2013, the White House's Office of Science and Technology Policy issued the *S&T Roadmap*. Building upon the *National Strategy for Biosurveillance*, the *Roadmap* identifies biosurveillance capability needs and key research and development priorities, including those related to integration. For example, the roadmap proposes the development of a national, interagency biosurveillance data- sharing framework that integrates data and information from disparate sources, as well as the development of tools that enhance the efficient manipulation of large data sets, including social media.

EXAMPLE OF A BIOLOGICAL EVENT MONITORED BY THE NATIONAL BIOSURVEILLANCE INTEGRATION CENTER

Ebola virus disease (EVD)

Since late 2013, the World Health Organization (WHO) has reported a cumulative over 27,000 suspected, probable, and confirmed cases of EVD and over 11,000 related deaths as of June 2015. The vast majority of cases have been in West Africa, but there have also been cases in the United States. Eleven cases of EVD have been treated in the U.S., of which 9 recovered and 2 patients died. Of the 11 cases, 9 were presumed to have been contracted in West Africa and 2 were presumed to have been contracted at a Texas hospital by nurses treating an infected patient.

EVD symptoms typically develop 2 to 21 days after exposure to Ebola virus. Symptoms include fever, headache, joint and muscle aches, impaired liver and kidney function, stomach pain, and death. Although the WHO has classified the West African EVD epidemic as a Public Health Emergency of International Concern, the outbreak is considered to be unlikely to significantly affect U.S. public health.

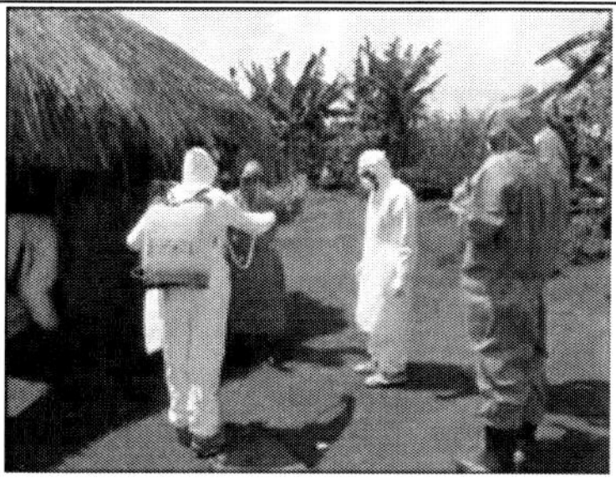

Source: National Biosurveillance Integration Center, Centers for Disease Control and Prevention (photo). | GAO 15-793

NBIC's Roles, Responsibilities, and Governance

As shown in table 2, the 9/11 Commission Act outlines certain requirements for NBIC. Drawing upon these requirements as well as the July 2012 *NBIC Strategic Plan*, we identified three main roles that NBIC, as a federal-level biosurveillance integrator, must carry out to achieve the duties and outcomes described by NBIC's authorizing legislation. Senior NBIC officials agreed that these three roles are consistent with the center's responsibilities. These roles are not mutually exclusive and can reinforce one other. For example, NBIC's efforts as an Innovator might result in the in the development of data that could enhance its role as an Analyzer by providing the center with another dataset to review.

NBIC is governed by the NBIC Advisory Board, which serves as the Assistant Secretary–level body for coordination and communication regarding integrated biosurveillance among the interagency biosurveillance community.[12] According to the board's November 2013 charter, the Advisory Board is to ensure input on and timely resolution of NBIC operational, programmatic, and scientific issues affecting the broader biosurveillance community, and to provide recommendations to DHS to assist in achieving NBIC goals. The board is to meet at least twice a year and is to be chaired by DHS's Chief Medical Officer, with a cochair that is to be rotated annually among the federal partners by a majority vote. The NBIC Advisory Board members are to provide formal recommendations to the Advisory Board Chair and Cochair on: (1) identifying, prioritizing, and addressing NBIC and other appropriate operational and programmatic needs; (2) reviewing draft guidance and other supporting documents related to national biosurveillance strategy and policy, as appropriate; and (3) improving communications and collaboration among local, state, tribal, territorial, and federal interagency partners. The NBIC Interagency Working Group is to provide support and respond to taskings from the Advisory Board to assist in addressing NBIC operational, programmatic, and scientific issues. The working group is to consist of senior-level federal officials from NBIS member departments and agencies and the Executive Office of the President who are authorized to make recommendations on behalf of their organizations. Each agency is to have at least one working group member, but can have more based on the relevance to their missions of the topics to be covered by the working group or subworking groups. The working group is to meet as needed, but generally more frequently than the Advisory Board, according to NBIC officials.

Table 2. Examples of the National Biosurveillance Integration Centers' (NBIC) Responsibilities from the 9/11 Commission Act of 2007 Organized by Biosurveillance Integrators Roles Identified by GAO

Role	Examples of NBIC responsibilities from the 9/11 Commission Act
Analyzer: Use technological tools and subject matter expertise to develop shared situational awareness by creating meaningful new insights from disparate datasets and information that could not be gleaned in isolation	• Consolidate data from all relevant surveillance systems maintained by member agencies across human, animal, and plant domains • Use an information technology (IT) system with the best available statistical and other analytical tools to identify and characterize biological events of national concern in as close to real time as practical • Receive and consider other relevant homeland security information, as appropriate
Coordinator: Bring together multi-disciplinary partners across interagency organizations to enhance understanding of new or potential biological events, such as through the collaborative development of products and services	• Oversee the development and operation of the National Biosurveillance Integration System (NBIS) • Alert NBIS member agencies as well as public health agencies of state, local, and tribal governments (in coordination with or through member agencies) of incidents that could develop into a biological event of national concern • Provide support for personnel from member agencies with sufficient expertise to analyze and interpret data
Innovator: Facilitate the development of new tools, technology, and approaches to address gaps in biosurveillance integration	• Provide the infrastructure for integration, including IT systems • Seek private sources of surveillance when such sources would enhance coverage of gaps • Monitor the availability and appropriateness of surveillance systems used by the center and those systems that could enhance biological situational awareness or the overall performance of the center

Source: GAO analysis of the 9/11 Commission Act and the *NBIC Strategic Plan*. | GAO-15-793

Example of a Biological Event Monitored by the National Biosurveillance Integration Center

Measles in the United States

From December 2014 through February 2015, state and local health departments reported 171 measles cases across 20 states and the District of Columbia. Most of these cases had been associated with an ongoing outbreak associated with Disneyland theme parks in California.

Measles is a highly contagious viral illness that can spread rapidly in communities without proper vaccination. Symptoms include high fever, cough, runny nose, watery eyes, rash, and death. Measles was officially declared eliminated in the U.S. in 2000 and cases in the U.S. have primarily the result of international travel to countries experiencing outbreaks. Outbreaks in the U.S. have persisted mainly due to the increase in unvaccinated people.

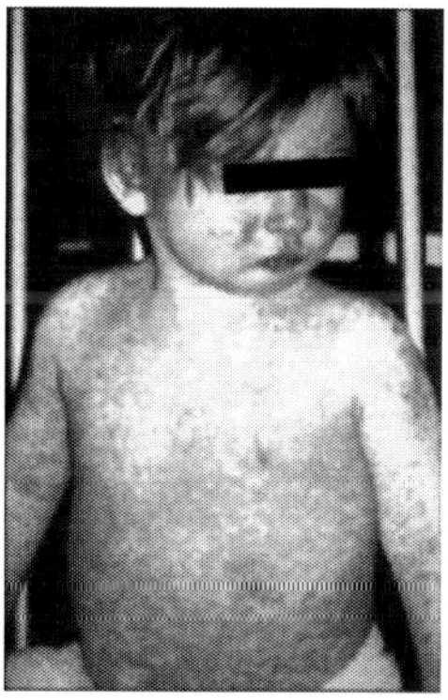

Source: National Biosurveillance Integration Center, Centers for Disease Control and Prevention (photo). | GAO 15-793

Interagency Biosurveillance Community

The NBIS is a consortium of federal partners that was established to rapidly identify and monitor biological events of national concern and to collect; analyze; and share human, animal, plant, food, and environmental biosurveillance information with NBIC.[13] The NBIS community predated the enactment of the 9/11 Commission Act. Beginning in 2004, DHS coordinated the NBIS community and developed an information technology (IT) system to integrate other agencies' biosurveillance information, an effort that was moved among several DHS directorates, including DHS's Science and Technology Directorate. In 2007, DHS created the Office of Health Affairs, headed by the DHS Chief Medical Officer, to lead DHS's biodefense activities and provide timely incident- specific guidance for the medical consequences of disasters. At that time, DHS placed the responsibility for coordinating the NBIS in the Office of Health Affairs. Shortly after that, the 9/11 Commission Act created NBIC and gave it responsibility for coordinating the NBIS. NBIC has remained in the Office of Health Affairs since that time.

EXAMPLE OF A BIOLOGICAL EVENT MONITORED BY THE NATIONAL BIOSURVEILLANCE INTEGRATION CENTER

Porcine epidemic diarrhea virus (PEDv)

Since Spring 2013, there have been 11,364 confirmed samples of PEDv from 35 states as of April 2015. As a result, 5 countries and the European Union issued trade restrictions against U.S. swine imports, some of which have since lifted those restrictions. Hog and pig farming is a multi-billion dollar industry. However, despite earlier predictions, the economic decline due to PEDv has not been as drastic as predicted.

PEDv is a highly infectious virus specific to swine and does not affect humans or other species. Symptoms in pigs include diarrhea, vomiting, and anorexia, and is particularly deadly to young pigs. In June 2014, the U.S. Department of Agriculture issued a Federal Order requiring mandatory reporting of all novel swine enteric coronavirus diseases, including PEDv.

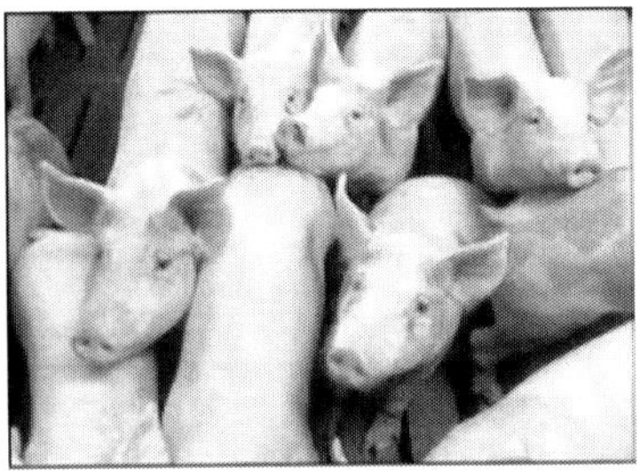

Source: National Biosurveillance Integration Center, U.S. Department of Agriculture (photo). | GAO 15-793

NBIC officials identified 14 federal partners that compose the NBIS. These departments and agencies, which are all signatories to the November 2013 charter of the NBIC Advisory Board, are DHS; the Departments of Agriculture (USDA), Commerce, Defense (DOD), Energy, Health and Human Services (HHS), the Interior (DOI), Justice, State, Transportation (DOT), and Veterans Affairs (VA); the Environmental Protection Agency (EPA); the United States Postal Service; and the Office of the Director of National Intelligence (ODNI). The 9/11 Commission Act outlines a number of responsibilities for member agencies.[14] For example, the member agencies are to use their best efforts to integrate biosurveillance information into NBIC and connect their biosurveillance data systems to the NBIC data system under mutually agreed protocols. Further, per the act, member agencies are to provide personnel to NBIC under an interagency personnel agreement and consider the qualifications of such personnel necessary to provide human, animal, and environmental data analysis and interpretation support to NBIC.

We surveyed and interviewed officials from 19 federal departments and their component agencies across 13 of the 14 departments and agencies that compose the NBIS.[15] On the basis of their roles and responsibilities related to biosurveillance, we categorized the NBIS partner agencies into three groups:

- ***Primary biosurveillance agencies:*** Primary biosurveillance agencies have major biosurveillance mission responsibilities that include collecting or analyzing biosurveillance information for the purposes of detecting, monitoring, or responding to biological events. These agencies generate information and develop subject matter expertise in pursuit of their missions that is directly relevant to disease detection and monitoring. In addition, they consume information from multiple sources—including nonfederal sources—to help achieve their missions. Examples of primary biosurveillance agencies include HHS's Centers for Disease Control and Prevention (CDC) and USDA's Animal and Plant Health Inspection Service (APHIS). Eleven of the 19 NBIS partners we interviewed and surveyed are primary biosurveillance agencies.
- ***Support biosurveillance agencies:*** Support biosurveillance agencies do not have missions that directly involve disease detection and monitoring; however, they collect data and information or have subject matter expertise that may be useful to efforts to detect, monitor, or respond to biological events. For example, the Department of Commerce's National Oceanic and Atmospheric Agency collects

meteorological data that may be used by NBIC to help inform the officials about progression of an outbreak based on weather patterns. Five of the 19 NBIS partners we interviewed and surveyed are support biosurveillance agencies.

See Appendix I for additional information on Figure 1.

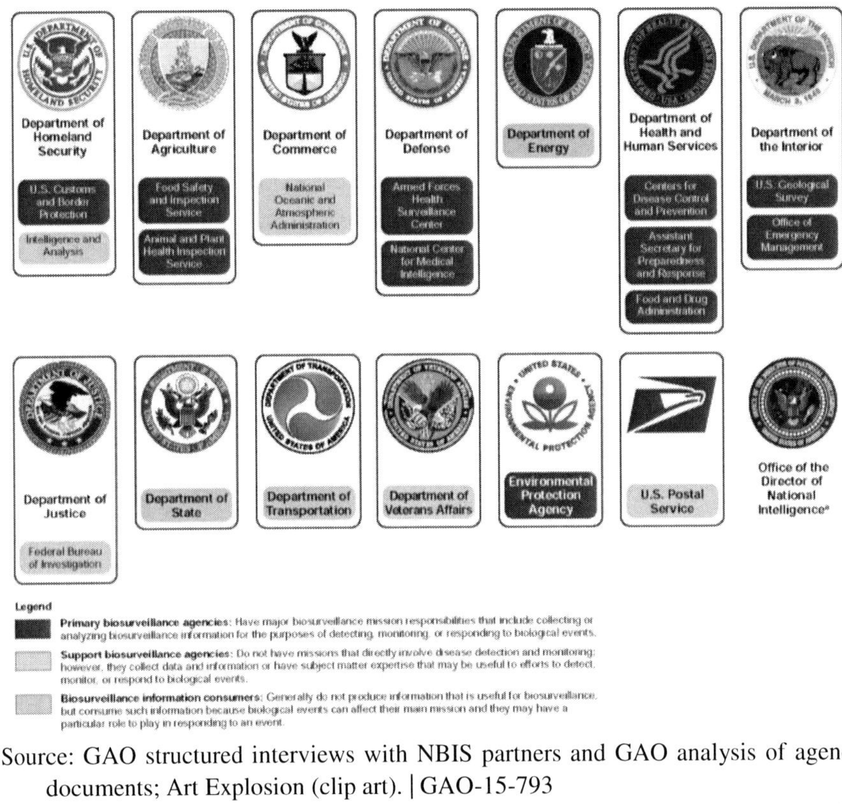

Source: GAO structured interviews with NBIS partners and GAO analysis of agency documents; Art Explosion (clip art). | GAO-15-793

[a] The Office of the Director of National Intelligence (ODNI) is represented on the National Biosurveillance Integration Center (NBIC) Advisory Board and NBIC Interagency Working Group. However, NBIC's relationship with the intelligence community is run through the Department of Homeland Security's Office of Intelligence and Analysis (I&A), according to our discussions with ODNI, NBIC, and I&A. In addition, NBIC's relationship with ODNI was new at the time of this review, and NBIC had not established direct relationships with ODNI. As a result, we did not include ODNI in additional interviews and the survey.

Figure 1. Biosurveillance Responsibilities of the National Biosurveillance Integration System Partners.

- ***Biosurveillance information consumers:*** Biosurveillance information consumers generally do not have missions that directly involve disease detection and monitoring and generally do not produce information that is useful for biosurveillance. However, they consume such information because biological events can affect their main mission and they may have a particular role to play in responding to an event. For example, officials from DOT stated that their department consumes biosurveillance information because biological events can affect the national transportation system and transporting people and items through a contaminated area can further exacerbate a biological event. Three of the 19 NBIS partners we interviewed and surveyed are biosurveillance information consumers.

Figure 1 and appendix I describe the missions and biosurveillance responsibilities of the 19 NBIS partners we interviewed and surveyed.

NBIC Has Activities that Support Integration, but Faces Challenges that Limit its Ability to Enhance the National Biosurveillance Capability

NBIC Compiles Information on Key Global Biological Events, but Faces Challenges Applying Statistical and Analytical Tools to Create New Meaningful Information

To fulfill its Analyzer role, NBIC develops a variety of products to enable early warnıng and enhance situational awareness of biological events, but the center faces challenges related to its ability to develop products that contribute meaningful information and has difficulty obtaining biosurveillance data.

NBIC's Analyzer Role Products and Activities

NBIC's efforts to fulfill its Analyzer role include a variety of products and activities designed to enable early warning and shared situational awareness. As part of its daily analytic process, NBIC analysts review two main types of information: (1) open source, such as media reports, foreign, national, state, and local government agency websites, and industry and professional association reports and websites, and (2) partner-provided. First, to identify relevant open-source information, NBIC uses both automated and manual methods. For example, in addition to conducting manual searches of media, NBIC analysts also access commercial open source data feeds such as HealthMap and DOD's National Center for Medical Intelligence's (NCMI) Arkham data feeds, which provide open-source information in more than 80 languages that are translated automatically into English.[16] Second, NBIC also relies on finished analytical products from NBIS partners, which may be obtained directly from partners or are available publically on agency websites. These products are usually received or obtained as written reports that represent the agency's analysis and interpretation of the raw data that it collects on a routine basis or for a specific event. NBIC analysts may also make requests for information to NBIS partners for additional information.

NATIONAL BIOSURVEILLANCE INTEGRATION CENTER (NBIC) DAILY ANALYTIC PROCESS WITH GENERAL TIME FRAMES

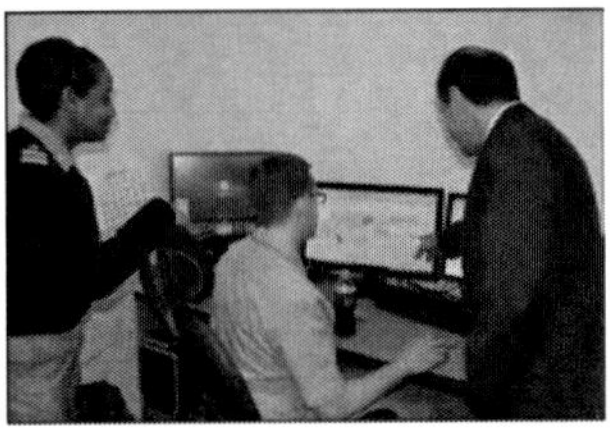

- ***24 hours a day*: Department of Homeland Security's Office of Health Affairs Watch Desk evaluates open- source biosurveillance information using a variety of tools and sources, which will inform the development of future products. NBIC analysts review watch desk information and reports from federal partners to identify items of potential significance.
- ***Late morning***: Analysts conduct a daily internal NBIC discussion to determine items of significance and decide additional actions that are required.
- ***Afternoon***: The *Daily Biosurveillance Review* is distributed to internal recipients including agency liaisons, and serves as a tool that generates a record of what was known, at what time, and from what source.

- ***Late afternoon***: Monitoring List is distributed via e-mail to federal partners and other domestic and international stakeholders to update them on items being monitored, as well as other reports published by NBIC.

Source: GAO analysis of National Biosurveillance Integration Center policies and procedures. | GAO 15-793

NBIC produces a variety of regular products to enable early warning and enhance situational awareness, including its daily Monitoring List, Biosurveillance Event Reports, and Special Event Reports, as well as by responding to requests for information from its partners. NBIC's Monitoring List is a daily e-mail that contains brief summaries on acute, ongoing biological events of concern or interest to the NBIS partners. Biosurveillance Event Reports provide additional detail on specific events. For example, throughout 2015, NBIC produced such reports on the Middle East respiratory syndrome coronavirus, highly pathogenic avian influenza, Ebola virus disease, measles, and porcine epidemic diarrhea virus, among others. NBIC has also produced Special Event Reports at the request of state and local authorities in advance of mass gathering events, such as the Super Bowl and the Little League World Series. NBIC also responds to requests for information from the NBIS partners and other stakeholders.

NBIC's Challenges as an Analyzer

According to agency officials we spoke with and strategic documents we reviewed, NBIC faces challenges in implementing its Analyzer role, including its limited ability to develop products that contribute meaningful information to its partners and difficulty obtaining biosurveillance data.

Products that Provide New Meaningful Information

Primary biosurveillance agencies generally reported that NBIC's products do not provide them with meaningful information because those products contain information that they either already generate themselves or could obtain directly from other NBIS partners more quickly. As illustrated in figure 2, during our structured interviews, 8 of 11 primary biosurveillance agencies reported that NBIC products and activities help their agency identify potential or ongoing biological events (i.e., perception) to little or no extent. For example, officials from 2 of these agencies stated that much of the information in NBIC's products related to their respective domains do not inform their biosurveillance activities because this information generally originates from reports that their agencies release publically.

Further, officials from multiple agencies described information-sharing networks outside of their participation with NBIC that they use to pursue their missions, including integrating information across domains—such as animal and human health data. For example, officials from 10 of the 11 primary biosurveillance agencies reported during our structured interviews that they integrate biosurveillance information from both within and outside their respective domains. As illustrated by figure 3 and appendix II, the primary and support biosurveillance agencies reported that they directly obtain information that enhances their situational awareness (i.e., perception, comprehension, and projection) of biological events from many of the other federal agencies in the NBIS. As a result, partners reported that NBIC's products contain much information of which they are already aware or could access regardless of their participation with NBIC. For example, as illustrated by figure 3, EPA officials reported that their agency obtains information that enhances all three elements of situational awareness from seven agencies, including APHIS, CDC, and NBIC, among others. Further, EPA officials reported that they obtain information that enhances their comprehension and projection of biological events from DOI's Office of Emergency Management and NCMI.

However, agencies with more limited roles in biosurveillance, such as the biosurveillance support agencies and information consumers, had more favorable views on NBIC's products and activities. For example, as also illustrated by figure 2, 5 of the 8 biosurveillance support agencies and information consumers stated that NBIC's products and activities help their agencies identify potential or ongoing biological events (i.e., perception) to a moderate extent. Officials from some of these agencies reported that they leveraged NBIC products because their own agencies lacked time, capacity, or the infrastructure to regularly review disparate sets of information across multiple agencies and domains. For example, officials from a support biosurveillance agency reported that because the agency did not have the capacity to review all of the relevant biosurveillance information that it collected, NBIC's products filled a critical information gap in its intelligence. Some NBIS partners suggested that NBIC's reports might be useful for state and local entities that might not have access to the same breadth of information or the capacity to integrate biosurveillance information themselves.

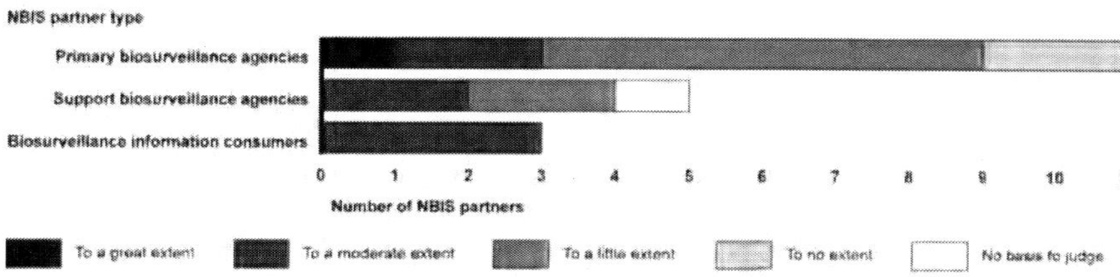

Source: GAO interview with NBIS partners. | GAO-15-793

Figure 2. National Biosurveillance Integration System (NBIS) Partner Views on the Extent to Which the National Biosurveillance Integration Center (NBIC) Enhances Their Perception of Biological Events.

Analytic Products and Activities of the National Biosurveillance Integration Center (NBIC)

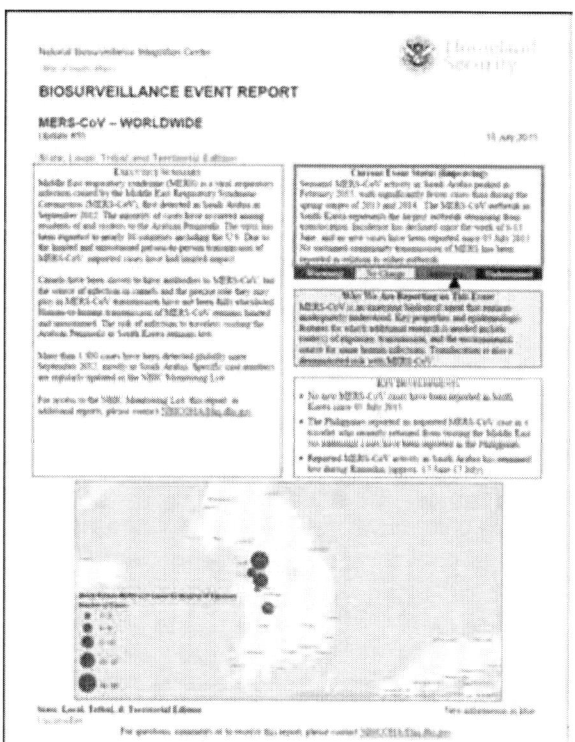

BIOSURVEILLANCE EVENT REPORT

MERS-CoV – WORLDWIDE

- **NBIC Monitoring List:** a daily e-mail to inform partners of new and ongoing events that NBIC is currently monitoring. These emails are sent to (1) federal; (2) state, local, tribal, and territorial; and (3) congressional users.
- **Biosurveillance Event Report:** a more detailed report focused on a specific event. These reports provide basic event details (e.g., pathogen, location, affected populations, and event progression) and describe interagency actions, among other things. These reports are distributed via e-mail as well as the Homeland Security Information Network, among others.
- **Special Event Report:** a report requested by government partners, such as state and local governments, to provide a public health assessment for a selected event.
- **Requests for Information:** biosurveillance information collection and gathering technique through analyst-to- analyst communications that can be submitted through the Department of Homeland Security's National Operations Center, e-mail, phone calls, or a biosurveillance information-sharing portal known as Wildfire.

Source: National Biosurveillance Integration Center, GAO analysis. | GAO 15-793

Further, as illustrated by figure 4, 5 of the 8 biosurveillance support agencies and information consumers stated that NBIC's products and activities help their agencies understand the nature and scope of emerging biological events (i.e., comprehension) to a great or moderate extent. Officials from these agencies generally stated that NBIC's products were easy to understand and provided useful context for events outside their scope of expertise. For example, officials from a support biosurveillance agency praised one of NBIC's Biosurveillance Event Reports on the recent outbreak of highly pathogenic avian influenza, which included information from CDC, APHIS, and USDA's Food Safety and Inspection Service (FSIS) on how the disease will affect the food chain, if it could cross to the human population, and what information is known locally.

The size of the circle for an NBIS partner reflects the number of times other primary and support biosurveillance agencies identified that agency as an information source that enhances situational awareness of a biological event. See Appendix II for additional information on Figure 3.

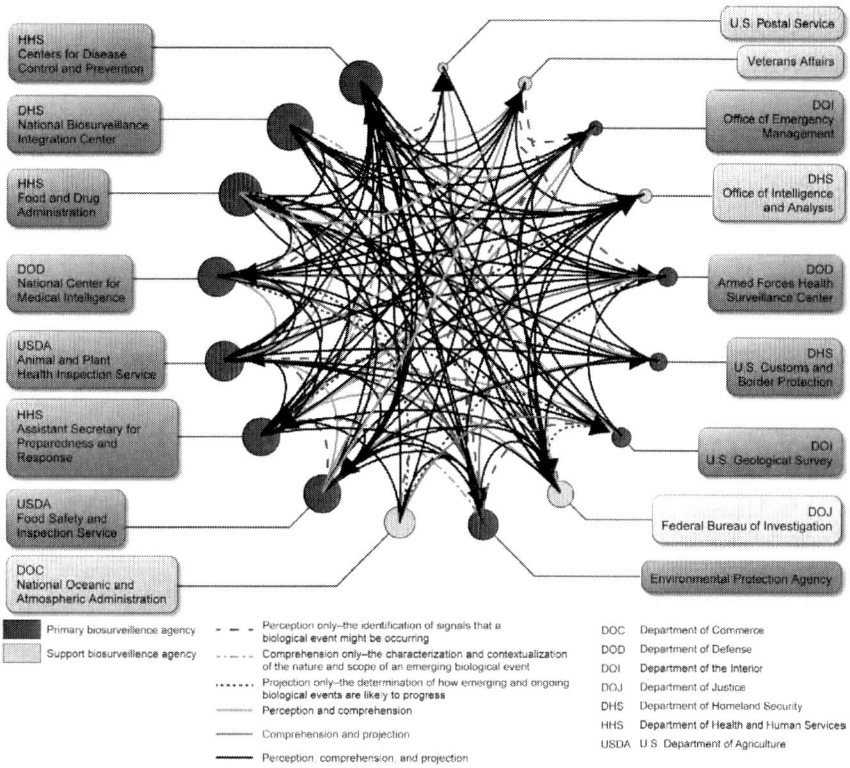

Source: GAO survey of NBIS partners. | GAO-15-793

The size of the circle for an NBIS partner reflects the number of times other primary and support biosurveillance agencies identified that agency as an information source that enhances situational awareness of a biological event.

Figure 3. Primary and Support Biosurveillance Agencies' Sources for Information That Enhances Situational Awareness of Biological Events.

Regardless of their role in biosurveillance, partners noted that NBIC's products and activities do not generally contribute new meaning or analysis—that is, insights that cannot be gleaned in isolation. For example, as shown in figure 5, 10 NBIS partners stated that NBIC's products and activities enhance their agencies' ability to carry out their biosurveillance roles and responsibilities to little or no extent, 4 responded to a moderate extent, and 5 responded that they did not have a basis to judge.[17] Generally, partners that responded to little or no extent noted that NBIC products and activities do not, for example, identify trends and patterns or describe potential impacts of a biological event. For example, officials from a primary biosurveillance agency stated that NBIC's products and activities do not "connect the dots" between dissimilar information, provide novel synthesis of information, or recommend possible courses of action.

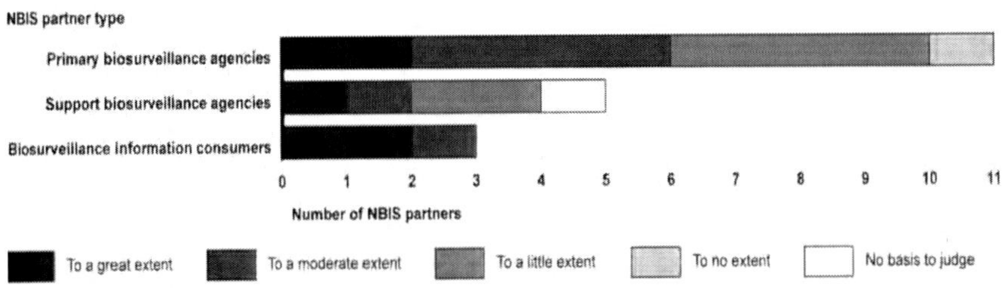

Source: GAO interviews with NBIS partners. | GAO-15-793

Figure 4. National Biosurveillance Integration System (NBIS) Partner Views on the Extent to Which the National Biosurveillance Integration Center (NBIC) Enhances Their Comprehension of Biological Events.

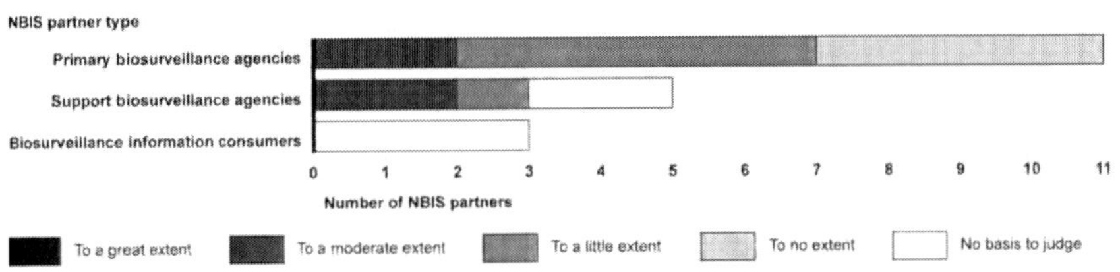

Source: GAO interviews with NBIS partners. | GAO-15-793

Figure 5. National Biosurveillance Integration System (NBIS) Partner Views on the Extent to Which the National Biosurveillance Integration Center (NBIC) Enhances Their Agency's Ability to Carry Out Its Biosurveillance Roles.

Further, as shown in figure 6, 11 of the 19 NBIS partners stated that NBIC's products and activities help their agencies understand how emerging and ongoing biological events are likely to progress into the near future (i.e., projection) to little or no extent. Officials noted that forecasting and projection are inherently difficult, but suggested that NBIC could develop other kinds of analysis that would be useful for the projection element of situational awareness. For example, officials from a primary biosurveillance agency suggested that NBIC could integrate more data and information from other DHS components into its reports, which would help to provide a homeland security perspective on biological events. Officials from another agency stated that NBIC could combine information across multiple domains on a local disease outbreak with known travel and weather patterns to predict how a disease might spread.

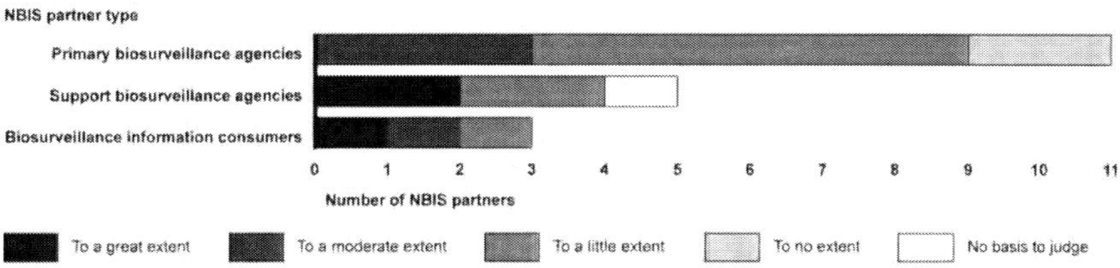

Source: GAO interviews with NBIS partners. | GAO-15-793

Figure 6. National Biosurveillance Integration System (NBIS) Partner Views on the Extent to Which the National Biosurveillance Integration Center (NBIC) Enhances Their Understanding of How Biological Events Are Likely to Progress (i.e., Projection).

NBIC officials stated that the center is working to improve its products and its ability to contextualize the information it collects from open sources, and has sought partner input to do so. For example, beginning in late June 2015, partly on the basis of feedback the center received from its November 2014 Federal Stakeholder Survey, NBIC modified its daily Monitoring List to include an up-front summary that identifies the status of ongoing biological events as worsening, improving, unchanged, or undetermined. During our interviews with the NBIS partners, several agency officials suggested that the center make a similar change to this product because it would help them to more quickly scan the report to determine which events might be worth further examination. Although we are not able to analyze the effect this change had on partner views because the change took place after our interviews, it appears to be a positive step in response to one issue that partners raised. Further, NBIC officials noted that the center is also working to better integrate forecasts and projections into its products and activities. Specifically, NBIC is participating in a working group led by the Office of Science and Technology Policy to support the priorities articulated in the *S&T Roadmap* by developing a common interagency vision for specific federal capabilities and practical next steps leading to the application of reliable infectious disease forecasting models in decision-making processes.

Data Availability and Access

Data that NBIC could use to identify and characterize a biological event of national concern using statistical and analytical tools, as called for in the 9/11 Commission Act, are limited. Apart from searches of global news reports and other publically available reports generated by NBIS partners, NBIC has been unable to secure streams of raw data from multiple domains across the biosurveillance enterprise that would lend themselves to near-time quantitative analysis that could reveal unusual patterns and trends. NBIC acknowledged in its strategic plan that the data required to carry out its mission as envisioned in the 9/11 Commission Act either do not exist or are subject to a variety of information sharing challenges that make a large information technology-centered solution less feasible than originally imagined.

NBIC and NBIS partners noted that there were several kinds of data that could be useful for this kind of biosurveillance integration, but these data may not exist or may not be in a usable form. For example, EPA officials stated that under the existing statutory framework, the federal government does not collect real-time data on water quality and contamination from drinking water utilities. Instead, water systems report violations of drinking water standards to EPA on a quarterly basis. In addition, officials from CBP and DOI's U.S. Geological Survey (USGS) reported that there is a significant gap in the availability of animal health data, particularly data on wildlife disease, which makes it difficult to fully understand the dynamics of zoonotic diseases. NBIC officials also noted that other kinds of data are maintained in formats that make them difficult to analyze, such as paper health records. Further, the *S&T Roadmap* noted that many livestock health records are held by private industry and are not broadly accessible or standardized in a manner that would make such data usable.

In our survey, few—5 of 19—NBIS partners reported that they shared raw data with NBIC, and during structured interviews NBIS partners discussed a variety of challenges they faced in sharing certain data with NBIC.[18] Some agencies are reluctant to share their data with NBIC because they are unsure how the information will be used. For example, officials from a primary biosurveillance agency stated that the agency does not share some data with NBIC because sharing such information too broadly might have substantial implications on agricultural trade or public perception of safety. Further, officials from another primary biosurveillance agency noted that there is sometimes reticence to share information and data with components of DHS because, given the department's roles in law enforcement and national security, the information might be shared outside of the health security community in a way that lacks appropriate context and perspective.

Other agencies stated that they are unable to share data for regulatory or legal reasons, or because appropriately protecting the data would take too long. For example, officials from HHS's Food and Drug Administration (FDA) stated that their agency is unable to share some of its data on food and drug contamination because this information is confidential commercial information that FDA is restricted from sharing outside the agency. According to CDC officials, their agency receives electronic data from state, territorial, local, and tribal sources for a variety of programs and purposes that are covered by data use agreements that do not allow CDC to share the data outside the terms of those agreements and as allowed or required by applicable federal laws, such as the Privacy Act of 1974 and the Freedom of Information Act.[19] Pursuant to federal law and the terms of these agreements, CDC may share aggregated information as long as it protects an individual's privacy. However, according to CDC officials, some of these data cannot be shared without extensive, time- consuming work to appropriately redact the data to ensure that individuals may not be identified and that privacy is protected, which results in the release of the data being postponed to the point that the data are no longer actionable. Further, officials from VA noted that the Health Insurance Portability and Accountability Act of 1996 and its implementing regulations also restrict their ability to share some data because it requires appropriate safeguards to protect the privacy of personal health information, and sets limits and conditions on the uses and disclosures that may be made of such information without patient authorization.[20]

Concerns over data are a long-standing issue with NBIC and the federal biosurveillance integration mission. We have previously reported that scant availability of data throughout the federal government, a lack of trust, and partners' concerns over sharing sensitive information with NBIC were major barriers in NBIC's ability to obtain the data and other information that it needed to support data integration.[21] NBIC officials recognize that these barriers inhibit the ability of their partners to share some data with the center, but noted that they are trying to work with some of their partners to address these issues. For example, NBIC is currently developing a project with VA to determine how the center can use VA's data for biosurveillance purposes while ensuring that sensitive data are properly managed.

NBIC Has Developed Procedures to Coordinate with Biosurveillance Partners, but Faces Limited Participation and Provision of Partner Personnel

To fulfill its Coordinator role, NBIC has established procedures that occur daily, weekly, and as emerging or significant biological event occur, but the center faces challenges related to participation of NBIS partners in the center's activities, the provision of partner personnel to NBIC, and competing structures for convening NBIS partners.

NBIC's Coordinator Role Products and Activities

NBIC's efforts to fulfill its Coordinator role with its partners includes a variety of interactions and established procedures that occur daily, weekly, and as emerging or significant biological events occur, including the NBIS Protocol, daily and weekly calls, by moderating an information sharing portal, and jointly developed products.

- **NBIS Protocol**: A mechanism that brings federal partners together to provide information sharing on an emerging or significant biological event through a short-notice teleconference, the protocol is meant to accelerate the ability to characterize an event as rapidly as possible and seeks to gather the scientific and medical communities of interest to assess the biological threat. The protocol is activated at the request of any federal NBIS partner, or the White House, when a situation meets one of the thresholds previously established by the NBIS partners.[22] Participation in NBIS Protocol Calls is not mandatory, and an NBIS partner may choose to opt out based on the announced subject of the call. NBIC exercises the protocol two times a year. According to NBIC officials, the protocol has been activated once since fiscal year 2012, in April 2013 to discuss both the avian flu in China (H7N9) and Middle Eastern respiratory syndrome.
- **Daily Calls:** NBIC's Daily Analysts' Call is a daily internal teleconference in which NBIC analysts discuss information and analytic insights from the previous day, but all NBIS partners may call in.
- **Biweekly Calls:** Until recently NBIC hosted a Weekly Reporting Call to present and discuss the most significant biosurveillance events from the previous week. In response to feedback the center received from

its November 2014 Federal Stakeholder Survey, NBIC changed the format of the weekly call in January 2015 to a biweekly call with a rotating responsibility among the NBIS partners to provide a featured speaker on a relevant issue, as well as an opportunity to pose questions to NBIC and the other partners on ongoing or potential biological events.

- **Wildfire Web-Based Information-Sharing Portal:** Wildfire is a tool used and governed by the Biosurveillance Indications and Warnings Analytic Community, a self-governing interagency body composed of federal officials who are actively responsible for pursuing a biosurveillance mission.[23] The portal is housed within the National Center for Medical Intelligence. Federal officials who are actively responsible for pursuing a biosurveillance mission can share information about potentially significant biological events on Wildfire. According to NBIC officials, NBIC analysts routinely use the portal. In addition, as the moderator since August 2013, NBIC ensures that questions posed by officials across the interagency are answered in a timely manner.
- **Jointly-Developed Products**: NBIC also brings together its multidisciplinary partners to develop joint products that enhance understanding of new or potential biological events. For example, NBIC coordinated with APHIS to facilitate a study by DHS's Homeland Infrastructure Threat and Analysis Center that modeled the potential biological and economic impacts of the Kudzu bug, a pest that presents a potential risk to the U.S. soybean crop if pesticide applications failed. NBIC has also developed joint classified intelligence products developed by DHS's Office of Intelligence and Analysis by, for example, describing the scope and context of a biological agent in these products.

NBIC's Challenges as a Coordinator

According to agency officials we spoke with and strategic documents we reviewed, NBIC faces challenges that affect its ability to implement its Coordinator role, including the limited participation of NBIS partners in NBIC activities, limited provision of partner personnel to NBIC, and competing structures for convening NBIS partners.

Coordinator Products and Activities of the National Biosurveillance Integration Center (NBIC)

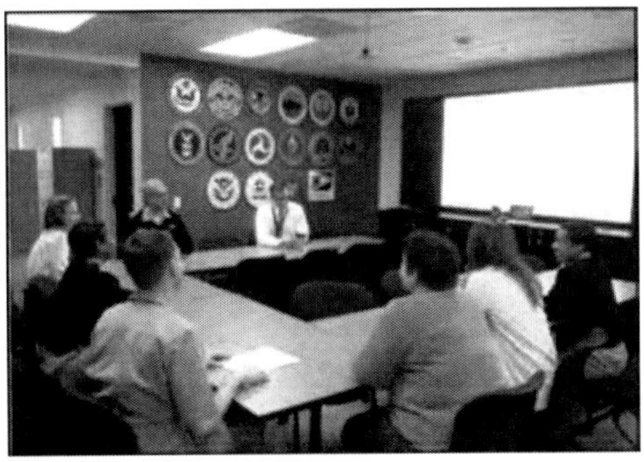

- **National Biosurveillance Integration System (NBIS) Protocol:** a mechanism that brings federal partners together on a short-notice teleconference to provide information sharing on an emerging or significant biological event.
- **Daily Analysts' Call:** a daily teleconference in which NBIC analysts and other participants discuss newly identified potential and active hazards.
- **Bi-weekly Reporting Call:** NBIC hosts the Interagency Biosurveillance Presentation Series bi-weekly via teleconference with NBIS Partners presenting and discussing biosurveillance project findings of interest.
- **Wildfire portal:** an encrypted interagency information-sharing portal— housed within the National Center for Medical Intelligence—through which participating entities can request information among a trusted subset of interagency subject matter experts within the federal biosurveillance community.
- **Jointly Developed Products:** NBIC brings together its multidisciplinary partners to develop joint products that enhance understanding of new or potential biological events.

Source: GAO analysis of NBIC policies and procedures. | GAO 15-793

Limited Participation

Although NBIC has implemented its Coordinator role through a variety of interactions and procedures, partner participation in key NBIC activities has generally been limited. For example, as shown in figure 7, about half of the NBIS partners reported in our survey that they regularly participated in NBIC's Weekly Reporting Calls (9 of 19) during the time period between August 2012 and December 2014, and even fewer reported regularly participating in the Daily Analyst Calls (2 of 19). Some of the agencies that reported not regularly participating in the daily and weekly calls are primary biosurveillance agencies that are generally considered to be among the lead generators of biosurveillance information in their respective domains. Officials from one of these agencies noted that much of the information presented during the daily and weekly calls was already provided in the daily Monitoring List e-mail, and therefore provided relatively little new information.

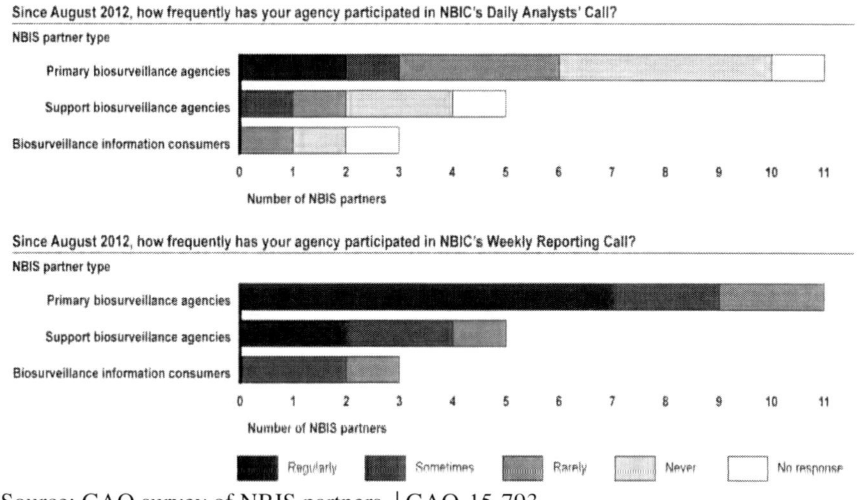

Source: GAO survey of NBIS partners. | GAO-15-793

Note: Because the format of weekly call changed in January 2015 during the course of our review, we asked survey respondents to identify the frequency with which they participated in the weekly call for the time period between August 2012 and December 2014.

Figure 7. National Biosurveillance Integration System (NBIS) Partners That Reported Participating in the National Biosurveillance Integration Center's (NBIC) Daily and Weekly Calls.

The *National Strategy for Biosurveillance* notes that in a reduced resources environment, it is important to pursue activities that add value for all participants, and officials across the NBIS noted that the modification to the weekly call was a positive step. For example, officials from a primary biosurveillance agency stated that the change provided them with an opportunity to advertise the services their agency provides. Officials from another primary biosurveillance agency noted that the new presentation-focused format is more likely to benefit all partners across the NBIS. NBIC officials stated that they plan to request feedback from the partners in the future on the new format of these calls to determine what, if any, additional changes are needed.

Limited Provision of Partner Personnel

Another challenge faced by NBIC concerns its ability to obtain personnel from its partners as originally envisioned in the 9/11 Commission Act. NBIC officials told us that effective biosurveillance depends on subject matter experts to interpret events and place them in context. Although all of the NBIS partners provide key points of contact for NBIC, few (3 of 19) partners currently provide a dedicated liaison as of July 2015. Officials across the NBIS partners provided various reasons for why their agencies did not provide a liaison. For example, officials from one primary biosurveillance agency stated that for their agency, and likely other agencies as well, it is difficult to provide personnel to NBIC on a full- or part-time basis because of their own resource constraints. Further, officials from a support biosurveillance agency noted that the lack of clarity about NBIC's value to its partners is a barrier to providing the center with detailees.

In order to obtain more personnel from its partners, NBIC has agreed to partially fund some of the liaisons. For example, according to NBIC officials, the center already funds liaisons from VA, DOI, and USDA's APHIS and is working to establish a liaison with CDC. According to NBIC, liaisons have provided great benefit to the center such as by providing special knowledge of their agency's roles and areas of responsibility and providing NBIC with the critical ability to reach-back into their respective agency or department. According to the officials, NBIC would like to more fully leverage the capabilities of its partners and obtain a liaison from each NBIS partner; however, budget constraints currently prohibit NBIC from obtaining fully funded liaisons from each partner.

Competing Structures for Convening Partners

Federal partners noted that they were unclear about the differences between two of the major structures used for convening federal stakeholders to discuss emerging biological events. The NBIS Protocol, as previously identified, is managed by NBIC, while the other, the Biological Assessment Threat Response (BATR) Protocol, is managed by the White House's National Security Council Staff. According to the *NBIC Strategic Plan*, the BATR Protocol is a national-level interagency consultation process with mid-to-high level decision makers that is designed to achieve coordinated action and desired outcomes to prevent, protect from, and respond to high-consequence bioterrorism and biosecurity threats.[24] According to NBIC, each of the protocols is designed to serve a different purpose for a different set of participants according to their respective roles in the recognition of, and response to, a biological event. The NBIS Protocol is a mechanism to bring together federal analysts and operators for information sharing early in a biological event's discovery and development phase; whereas the BATR Protocol is designed to enable the most senior level of federal leadership to achieve situational awareness to effectively coordinate available resources for incident response. However, although we did not ask a specific question about the two protocols in our structured interviews, about a quarter of the NBIS partners (5 of 19) we interviewed were unclear about the differences between the two protocols. For example, in structured interviews, officials from two of the agencies noted that the protocols appeared to serve the same purpose or were attended by the same officials.

NBIC Has Efforts Under Way to Develop New Biosurveillance Tools, but Faces Challenges Prioritizing Development Efforts in a Limited Resource Environment

To fulfill its Innovator role, NBIC has funded several pilot projects, sought new data sources, and made efforts to enhance its IT system, but faces challenges related to its limited resources and the varying needs of its partners.

NBIC's Innovator Role Products and Activities

NBIC's efforts to fulfill its role as an Innovator include conducting gap analyses, funding pilot projects that aim to develop new biosurveillance tools and technology, seeking new sources of data and information, and building its internal IT system. Beginning in September 2012, NBIC sought input from its federal partners to identify and prioritize biosurveillance capability gaps. According to NBIC officials, the gap analysis effort enabled NBIC to survey the biosurveillance community to identify any innovative pilot projects that NBIC could sponsor given its current resources and designed to provide broad support to the NBIS and other stakeholders, not only to NBIC. Specifically, NBIC requested that its partners identify existing capability gaps and suggest specific actions that would make progress toward a desired end state or outcome. In response, NBIC received 13 proposals from the NBIS partners, and then requested that partners prioritize the capability gaps for implementation. This prioritization was completed in April 2013. On the basis of the results, NBIC funded a pilot project to develop standardized methods of communicating the uncertainty of biosurveillance information. The project's aim was intended to help promote improved understanding when information is shared among biosurveillance analysts, leading to more rapid characterization and mitigation of disease outbreaks. The resulting product, which was completed in October 2014, provides biosurveillance analysts with procedures for selecting and applying uncertainty methods as well as a standardized format for reporting information.

The 2012 *NBIC Strategic Plan* also identified a number of pilot projects designed to assess the extent to which such projects could be adopted full-scale. According to the plan, each pilot project is intended to improve collaboration or information sharing. According to NBIC, these pilots are routinely assessed and evaluated to determine what is most helpful and effective, and those that prove successful will be integrated into normal operations, while those that are not will be discontinued. For example, NBIC has jointly funded the National Collaborative for Bio-Preparedness pilot project to develop a comprehensive, state-level system to analyze public health trends and detect emerging biological incidents by using data analytics and anomaly algorithms. Further, NBIC has also funded three pilot projects examining the feasibility of using open-source data from various social media applications in order to identify possible health trends. NBIC has completed two of these pilots and one is ongoing.

INNOVATOR PRODUCTS AND ACTIVITIES OF THE NATIONAL BIOSURVEILLANCE INTEGRATION CENTER (NBIC)

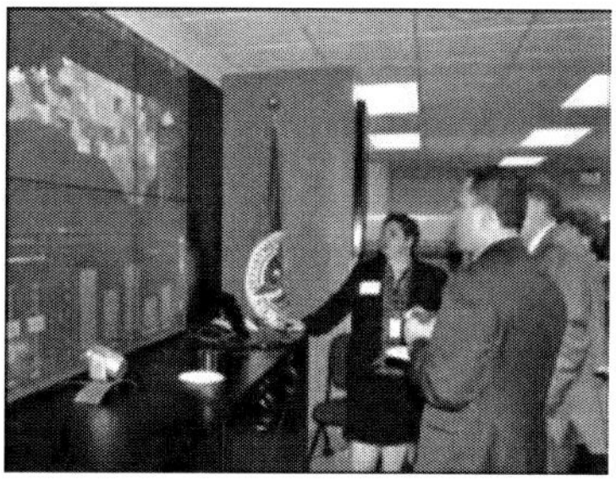

- **National Collaborative for Bio- Preparedness (NCB-Prepared):** a pilot project sponsored by NBIC and the University of North Carolina at Chapel Hill, among others. According to NBIC, a September 2014 prototype was capable of real-time analysis of health data in a geographic format, enabling users to search data, for example, on clinical symptoms and text within health records, using data from Emergency Medical Services, 911 phone calls, and Poison Control Centers. According to NBIC, this pilot program is intended to be offered to state and local governments and the private sector.
- **Social Media pilot projects:** NBIC has conducted several pilot projects to examine the extent that social media can augment existing biosurveillance detection and analysis. The pilot projects assessed the feasibility of using commercial and government off-the-shelf systems to aggregate social media information for biosurveillance. The most recent pilot, initiated in fiscal year 2012, funds the Department of Defense's Naval Surface Warfare Center to develop analytical techniques to improve the use of social media data for biosurveillance. NBIC plans to conclude the project at the end of fiscal year 2015, and transition the project's algorithms for operational use.

Source: National Biosurveillance Integration Center, GAO analysis. | GAO 15-793

NBIC has been seeking new sources of data and information in order to fulfill its mission for early warning and shared situational awareness of acute biological events, including data and information from other DHS components and NBIS partners, as well as classified information. First, in September 2013, NBIC analyzed the usefulness of department-wide absenteeism data from DHS's Office of the Chief Human Capital Officer, which could be an indicator of an emerging epidemic. Based on an analysis of 20 months of DHS workforce data from 2012 and 2013, the study concluded that absenteeism data could be a useful component in biosurveillance, as understanding differences between normal leave behavior and expected rises in leave behavior during peak flu seasons would help in establishing baseline values for comparison. In August 2014, NBIC, working with DHS's Science and Technology Directorate and Lawrence Livermore National Laboratory, evaluated the usefulness of DHS components' data systems as potential biosurveillance data sources. The assessment identified two Customs and Border Protection (CBP) databases as the most useful to NBIC's mission, and in June 2014, NBIC funded a part-time liaison to CBP's Office of Intelligence to determine the extent to which NBIC can use CBP databases for biosurveillance purposes.[25] Second, NBIC has also sought to obtain new sources of data from NBIS partners and other stakeholders. For example, as of July 2011, VA has provided NBIC a liaison to, among other responsibilities, identify ways NBIC can use VA's patient healthcare information to support its early detection and situational awareness mission. Finally, according to NBIC officials, the center has enhanced its process for analyzing intelligence information and reviews various intelligence sources to supplement, corroborate, or provide additional context to the biosurveillance items identified through other sources. For example, an NBIC intelligence analyst reviews all source intelligence information to identify potential topics of interest, such as indications of novel infectious disease or terrorism, and if necessary, reaches back to partners in the intelligence community for further information.

NBIC officials noted that the center's recent focus is on building its internal IT infrastructure, rather than pilot projects. For example, through its current Biofeeds project with the Pacific Northwest National Laboratory, NBIC is seeking to build a visual and text analytics capability that to enable the center to more effectively and efficiently identify relevant information in open source data. Officials also noted that NBIC is partnering with the Defense Threat Reduction Agency on the Biosurveillance Ecosystem project to build a collaborative analytic workbench for the center. Further, officials stated that NBIC has obtained an IT program manager as a detailee from the Transportation Security Administration to help build the center's internal IT program.

NBIC's Challenges as an Innovator

According to agency officials we spoke with and strategic documents we reviewed, NBIC faces challenges that affect its ability to implement its Innovator role, including its limited resources and the varying needs of partners.

Limited Resources

Although we did not ask a specific question about resource limitations, officials from 9 of the 19 NBIS partners identified it as a challenge NBIC faces in developing new biosurveillance tools and technology. From fiscal year 2012 through 2015, NBIC's budget ranged from $10 million to $13 million annually.[26] Officials from 2 primary biosurveillance agencies noted that NBIC's budget limits its ability to enhance its existing technology systems to invest in innovations such as disease event modeling. Further, officials from 3 primary biosurveillance agencies more generally expressed concerns regarding the imbalance between the size and nature of NBIC's mission, including its role as an innovator, and the resources that it had available to achieve it. NBIC officials stated they have never requested a budget increase, because their larger DHS office, the Office of Health Affairs, has experienced budget reductions, and an increase for NBIC would require a decrease for another program. However, NBIC officials noted that they would likely use any increase in its budget to help develop more analytical tools for itself and its partners.

Partners Have Varying Needs

Related to its limited resources, NBIC also faces challenges prioritizing its innovation efforts because its partners have diverse, and sometimes conflicting, needs. The *S&T Roadmap* noted that active collaboration for biosurveillance presents challenges because stakeholders have varying missions and roles. As previously noted, NBIC asked its partners to identify existing capability gaps. The 13 submissions covered a wide variety of biosurveillance issues and domains, such as wildlife disease surveillance, integration of pharmacy data, and analysis of Medicare claims data. However, although NBIC asked partners to prioritize the 13 submissions identified as existing capability gaps, the proposal that was selected had been ranked third by the partners, and officials from a primary biosurveillance agency stated that it was unclear why the higher ranking proposals were not selected. Further, officials from a primary biosurveillance agency suggested that NBIC conduct its own needs analysis to determine what tools and technology NBIC could invest in. NBIC officials noted that the third ranked proposal was selected because it was the highest ranked proposal that was "shovel ready", thereby allowing funding to be applied when funding was available, whereas the top two proposals were not. According to NBIC officials, future investments will be informed by the *S&T Roadmap*.

Biosurveillance Partners Expressed Skepticism about the Feasibility of NBIC's Mission

Although 13 of the 19 NBIS partners stated in our structured interviews that the concept of having a federal entity whose mission is to serve as the integrator of national biosurveillance information across agencies and disease domains is very or moderately important, some also expressed doubts about the feasibility and practicality of this mission. Specifically, although we did not specifically ask a question about the practicality of NBIC's mission, about a third of the NBIS partners (7 of 19) expressed skepticism and doubts about the feasibility of NBIC's mission, including whether federal integration of biosurveillance information could actually achieve early warning and situational awareness of biological events. Among the specific reasons officials cited for the skepticism was their uncertainty that the current model of biosurveillance integration was the most effective investment for strengthening the national biosurveillance capability. For example, officials from one agency noted that while the concept makes sense intuitively, there is no reliable evidence, such as a peer-reviewed study, that has confirmed the viability of the concept, nor has there been a large-scale biological threat that has been detected through integration; moreover, such a system—by virtue of its being federally-based—would lack timely detection and response capabilities because events occur at the local level. Officials from another agency questioned the feasibility of NBIC's mission because the data and technology that are currently available do not provide for the accurate projection of biological events or facilitate the provision of early warning. Additionally, an NBIC official told us that the ability to achieve early detection of emerging events—especially unexpected or novel events—is dubious because most of the tools and techniques used in surveillance rely on contrasting current conditions with known baseline trends and patterns, but as an event emerges, surveillance practitioners are not necessarily going to be focused on those patterns and trends until something prompts their attention. Moreover, when a biological event is novel, its patterns and trends are not yet known.

We have previously reported on skepticism on the part of some of the NBIS partners regarding the value of the federal biosurveillance mission as well as NBIC's role in that mission.[27] In our 2009 report, most of the NBIS partners we interviewed at that time expressed uncertainty about the value of participating in the NBIS or confusion about the purpose of NBIC's mission.[28] For example, officials from 1 of the partners stated that it was unsure whether NBIC contributed anything to the federal biosurveillance community that other agencies were not already accomplishing in the course of carrying out their biosurveillance-relevant missions. We, the NBIS partners, and other major stakeholders in the biosurveillance community acknowledge that no single problem limits NBIC's mission to integrate biosurveillance data. Rather, over the years, several long-standing problems have combined to inhibit the achievement of this mission as envisioned in the 9/11 Commission Act. Most notably, to operationalize the federal biosurveillance integration concept requires the simultaneous sharing and consideration of information from vastly disparate domains, including health, law enforcement, intelligence, and international partners. However, as noted in the *S&T Roadmap*, the sharing of this information is limited and is often not possible.

There Are a Range of Options for Addressing Biosurveillance Integration Challenges, and Each Has Associated Benefits and Limitations

The challenges previously described illustrate that NBIC faces significant obstacles in implementing its roles as a biosurveillance integrator as originally described in the 9/11 Commission Act. Below, we discuss options for policy or structural changes that could help better fulfill the biosurveillance integration mission. We identified these options and their benefits and limitations, on the basis of the roles of a federal-level biosurveillance integrator we identified in the 9/11 Commission Act, NBIC's strategic plan, and the perspectives of the NBIS partners obtained during our structured interviews. These options are not exhaustive, and some options could be implemented together or in part. In developing these options, we did not evaluate the financial implications of implementing each option, to the extent it is knowable, but we acknowledge they are likely to result in an increase, decrease, or shifting of funding based on the changes described.

Option 1: Reinforce NBIC's Analyzer Role

Under this option, NBIC would be provided with new authorities and resources designed to access additional public and private data sources and statistical and modeling tools to develop meaningful information. Although NBIC would continue monitoring for signals of global disease outbreaks using open-source data, as the center currently does, it would shift attention from daily reporting on known disease outbreaks around the world to bringing together diverse datasets to create and improve forecasts and identify hypothesis-driven underlying connections in seemingly unrelated datasets. This option may require new statutory authorities to ensure NBIC can obtain all available data and also may require changes or clarification of key applicable provisions of existing statutes and regulations. For example, some partners have cited the Health Insurance Portability and Accountability Act of 1996 and its implementing regulations related to protecting the privacy and security of personal health information as a reason for not sharing some biosurveillance information. To the extent that this option has the potential to result in a meaningful enhancement to the national biosurveillance capability, it may require significant new investments to do so—for example, to establish technology, systems, and legal frameworks that facilitate generation and sharing of data. Potential benefits and limitations of this option include the following:

Benefits

- **Developing meaningful information not otherwise available:** This option would address some of the challenges NBIC faces in implementing its Analyzer role, such as access to data from the NBIS partners, and would better position the center to develop meaningful information that could not be gleaned in isolation, potentially leading to earlier warning of emerging events and shared situational awareness.
- **Capitalize on new data sources and analysis techniques:** Focusing on providing the resources, infrastructure, and frameworks for data

sharing may provide the foundation to capitalize on future advancements in data analytics, including big data analysis and electronic health records, to mine data for emerging patterns.

Limitations

- **Uncertain need:** The probability that a disease event with significant national consequences occurring in such a way that it would be detected more quickly by overlaying various data streams and applying statistical and analytical tools to them is not known.
- **Uncertain data availability:** There may not be a significant amount of meaningful data available that is not already being provided to facilitate advanced analytical techniques. For example, although partners identified other potential data sources that could contribute to a more robust integration tool, such as water contamination and wildlife disease data, it is unknown whether such data could be collected and managed to make a meaningful contribution, and if they could, at what cost.
- **Unproven concept:** Even with access to more data, it is unclear whether a federal biosurveillance integrator would be able to identify patterns or connections that would lead to earlier warning of emerging events or reduce the time it takes to discover, prevent, or respond to a potentially catastrophic event, or that it would merit the associated costs. Finding patterns and trends without knowing specifically what to look for is challenging, and about a third of the NBIS partners (7 of 19) expressed skepticism and doubts about the feasibility of NBIC's mission, including whether federal integration of biosurveillance information could actually achieve early warning and situational awareness of biological events.
- **Unknown impact of earlier detection:** If NBIC were able to discern signals that gave warning of an emerging event, there is no guarantee that it would significantly decrease the amount of time it would take federal partners to confirm the warning and implement response actions.
- **Increased costs:** Creating the enterprise architecture both within NBIC and across the NBIS that would facilitate transfer and computer- aided analysis of data would likely require a significant investment in technology, as well as skilled personnel with data analytic, legal, and regulatory expertise. Although we have not

specifically assessed the costs of these options, such costs, at least in the near term, would likely exceed NBIC's current annual budget.

Option 2: Strengthen NBIC's Coordinator Role

Under this option, NBIC would be provided with greater authority for coordinating the federal biosurveillance enterprise. NBIC would be the operational agency accountable for overseeing the implementation of the *National Strategy for Biosurveillance*, drawing on the center's daily analytical capacity and the interagency governance infrastructure NBIC has already established. Responsibilities would include strategic oversight, such as helping to ensure consistency across the interagency for high-level policy and doctrine, and maintaining and creating the national strategy and related documents. Responsibilities could also include tactical coordination during national crises—drawing on the established NBIS Protocol and harmonizing it with parallel structures such as the BATR Protocol. Responsibilities could also include coordination to build interagency connections that result in shared analytical capacity, for which NBIC could draw upon and enhance established structures like Wildfire moderation and Daily Analysts; Calls. Potential benefits and limitations of this option include the following:

Benefits

- **Clear leadership:** This option would create clear leadership across the interagency for developing and implementing biosurveillance policy in general and in response to specific biological events, which may also encourage partners to more fully participate in NBIC activities, such as regularly attending NBIC's Daily Analysts' and Bi-weekly Reporting calls.
- **Better institutional connection:** NBIC officials have stated that the current liaisons have provided great benefit to the center. Ongoing interaction among more dedicated liaisons from various agencies may strengthen biosurveillance subject matter expertise and could enhance communication across all the agencies.
- **Routine, institutionalized channels to monitor for emerging trends and patterns:** Clarifying the federal integrator's role in routinely convening and drawing on the analytical capacity of the various pockets of federal expertise across the NBIS could enhance

the ability of NBIC to go beyond daily surveillance and monitoring activities to recognize connections and generate meaningful insights that may not be gleaned in isolation.

- **Enhanced accountability for implementing the *National Strategy for Biosurveillance*:** Formally vesting a federal entity with responsibility for leadership of the national biosurveillance enterprise would fill a longstanding need to institutionalize and create accountability for common goals and deliberate, results-driven, risk-based investment across the enterprise. Because the mission responsibilities and resources needed to develop a national biosurveillance capability are dispersed across a number of federal agencies, efforts could benefit from a focal point to provide sustained leadership that helps direct interagency efforts to invest in and implement new and existing programs in a way that ensures generation of meaningful data with the potential to discover emerging biological events with potentially catastrophic consequences.

Limitations

- **Role conflict:** Some of these responsibilities overlap with responsibilities that have historically been the purview of the National Security Council Staff, and legislative direction to assume these responsibilities could create more role conflict and confusion unless authority, roles, and responsibilities were very clearly designated.
- **Authority and legitimacy**: It may be difficult for an agency at NBIC's level to successfully influence decision making across the interagency. For example, discussions we had with some NBIS partners demonstrated that both DHS and NBIC have encountered and may continue to encounter issues with perceived legitimacy in the health security arena.

Option 3: Expand NBIC's Innovator Role

Under this option, NBIC would be provided with new authorities and resources to lead research and development investments of new tools and technology that would address gaps across the biosurveillance community. Responsibilities would include developing new analytical methods and IT systems, and seeking new sources of biosurveillance information, such as state, local, and private sources, including by developing new sources through systems like the National Collaborative for Bio-Preparedness. Efforts could be guided by the White House's *S&T Roadmap*, as well as other efforts to identify gaps in the national biosurveillance capability. For example, the *S&T Roadmap* identified 16 capability needs that are needed to strengthen biosurveillance, including those related to aberration detection; risk anticipation; threat identification and characterization; and information integration, analysis, and sharing. Potential benefits and limitations of this option include the following:

Benefits

- **New tools and technology:** NBIC could foster the development of tools and technology that benefit multiple federal partners and other members of the NBIS (e.g., state and local health agencies), thus enhancing the overall national biosurveillance capability. For example, the 2013 *S&T Roadmap* identified the need to strengthen detection by developing new modeling and ecological forecasting approaches that could enhance current ways of predicting disease outbreaks and determining likely impacts when a threat is detected. Specifically, this should be accomplished by developing methods that integrate traditional monitoring (i.e., pathogen, environmental, and health) with background data (i.e., meteorological and population dynamics).
- **Coordinate research and development efforts:** The *S&T Roadmap* notes that there are dozens, and possibly hundreds, of biosurveillance initiatives and pilot projects that have been implemented at local, state, regional, and national levels, NBIC would be well positioned to help coordinate and deconflict biosurveillance research and development across the interagency, which would help to avoid any unnecessary duplication, overlap, and fragmentation of effort. Further, the *S&T Roadmap* identifies 14 research priorities, many of which would benefit from coordination across the federal government, as well as with state, local, and private entities. For example, one of the research priorities is to develop multilateral communication mechanisms among the various levels of government and the private sector to enable timely decision making. Effectively addressing such a research priority would likely require the collaboration of multiple

federal and nonfederal partners, including HHS, USDA, and DHS, as well as healthcare providers and international partners, among others.

Limitations

- **Increased costs:** Although we have not specifically assessed the costs associated with the options, supporting the development of new tools and technology would likely exceed NBIC's current annual budget.
- **More research and development expertise:** Although NBIC has engaged in some pilot projects that develop tools and technology, a national integrator that focuses on innovation would likely need to acquire more expertise in research and development.
- **Significant restructuring:** In comparison with its other roles, NBIC's role as an Innovator is the least well defined in the 9/11 Commission Act, and NBIS partners noted that the center's current budget limits its ability to fulfill this role. Focusing attention on this role may represent a significant mission shift from the status quo, and may require very different sets of resources and procedures.

Option 4: Continue to Execute the 2012 *NBIC Strategic Plan*

In this option, NBIC would continue to implement the mission, goals, and objectives detailed in the August 2012 *NBIC Strategic Plan* or subsequent NBIS-approved updates. According to officials, NBIC is currently working on a mid-point review to assess progress made on meeting the goals described in the 2012 strategic plan and determine how best to accomplish priority activities and objectives by 2017, as identified by the NBIC Advisory Board and NBIC Interagency Working Group. Potential benefits and limitations of this option include the following:

Benefits

- **NBIC has made progress and may continue to do so:** Although most (10 of 19) federal partners stated that NBIC has limited impact on their ability to carry out their biosurveillance roles and responsibilities, 12 of 19 NBIS partners interviewed noted that NBIC has made improvements in its products, outreach, coordination, and other activities.[29] Further, in recent years, NBIC has been able to obtain or partially fund liaisons from other agencies. Establishing itself as a trusted and effective federal integrator with limited direct authority is a difficult task, and the center and its NBIS partners may merely need more time to evolve their roles and relationships to realize the full potential of the current NBIC as the federal biosurveillance integrator.

- **Some agencies currently find value in NBIC's products:** Agencies with more limited roles in biosurveillance, such as biosurveillance support agencies and information consumers, generally stated that they like NBIC's products because their own agencies do not have enough resources to review biosurveillance information across multiple agencies and domains. Further, NBIC officials noted that the center's products benefit some of their nonfederal stakeholders that have limited resources for biosurveillance, such as state, local, tribal, and territorial agencies. For example, as of July 2015, NBIC's daily Monitoring List e-mail is distributed to 338 individuals representing state, local, tribal, and territorial entities, including state departments of health and agriculture, fusion centers, and police departments.

Limitations

- **Data challenges:** NBIC will likely continue to face challenges in obtaining all the biosurveillance data it needs to effectively apply statistical and analytical tools to identify and characterize biological events of national concern in as close to real time as practicable, per requirements in the 9/11 Commission Act.
- **Partners remain skeptical of NBIC's value:** NBIC has implemented our recommendation to create a strategy, in partnership with the NBIS agencies, that better defines its mission and focus on other collaborative practices. Nevertheless, NBIS partners remain skeptical of NBIC's value. As previously shown in figure 5, few of the NBIS partners (4 of 19) we interviewed stated that NBIC's products and activities enhanced their agency's ability to carry out their biosurveillance roles and responsibilities. Further, as illustrated in figure 8, 8 of 19 NBIS partners we interviewed stated that NBIC is achieving its mission to little or no extent. It is unclear whether additional time or what additional actions will improve partners' experience with NBIC's overall value to the national biosurveillance capability.

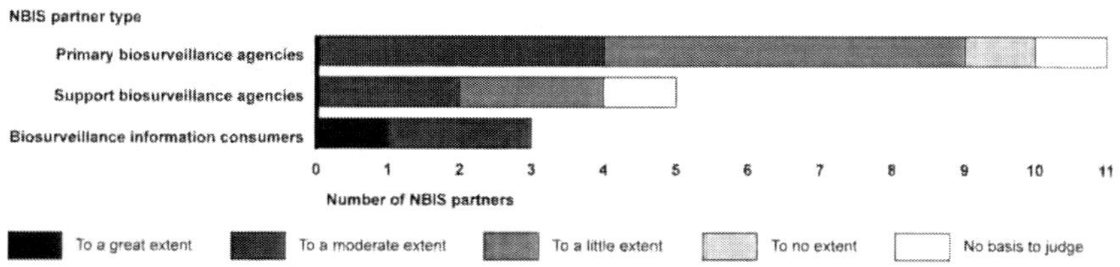

Source: GAO survey of NBIS partners. | GAO-15-793

Figure 8. National Biosurveillance Integration System (NBIS) Partner Views on the Extent to Which the National Biosurveillance Integration Center (NBIC) Is Achieving Its Biosurveillance Integration Mission.

Option 5: Repeal the NBIC Statute

In this option, national biosurveillance integration would not be pursued through NBIC. Consideration could be given to designating one of the other primary biosurveillance agencies as the federal biosurveillance integrator. Potential benefits and limitations of this option include the following:

Benefits

- **Cost savings:** Given that most federal partners stated that they integrate some biosurveillance information themselves and that NBIC has limited impact on their ability to carry out their biosurveillance roles and responsibilities, the cost of operating NBIC may not be worth its benefits.

Limitations

- **Officials report that a federal integrator is important:** Although federal partners generally thought that NBIC's products and activities did not provide meaningful new information, they largely thought that the concept of having a federal entity to integrate biosurveillance information across the federal government was important. Specifically, in our structured interviews, 13 of the 19 NBIS partners stated that the concept of having a federal entity whose mission is to serve as the integrator of national biosurveillance information across agencies and disease domains is very or moderately important.[30]

- **Potential loss of investment:** As previously noted, 13 of 19 NBIS partners stated that NBIC has made improvements in its products, outreach, coordination, and other activities. Defunding NBIC could create a loss of investment, institutional learning, and progress made toward developing a federal biosurveillance integrator, which may need more time to evolve to become effective.
- **Another integrator may experience similar challenges:** Even if one of the other primary biosurveillance agencies were designated as the federal biosurveillance integrator, that entity may still find it difficult to overcome organizational boundaries and engender agency cooperation, given that multiple agencies have key biosurveillance responsibilities.

AGENCY COMMENTS

We provided a draft of this report for review and comment to DHS and the 13 other departments and agencies that compose the NBIS—the Departments of Agriculture, Commerce, Defense, Energy, Health and Human Services, Interior, Justice, State, Transportation, and Veterans Affairs, as well as EPA, ODNI, and USPS. DHS provided written comments on September 16, 2015, which are summarized below. DHS, EPA, USPS, and the Departments of Agriculture, Interior, Health and Human Services, and Veteran's Affairs provided technical comments, which we considered and incorporated, where appropriate. The ODNI and the Departments of Commerce, Defense, Energy, Justice, State, and Transportation did not comment.

DHS expressed appreciation for our recognition of its progress fulfilling our prior recommendations, which were designed to enhance interagency collaboration. DHS also acknowledged the array of challenges detailed in this report, and noted some actions it is undertaking to try to address them. DHS noted that the report does not include nonfederal biosurveillance stakeholders in its scope, and posits that these stakeholders may find value in NBIC's current products. Although we cannot comment on the extent to which these nonfederal stakeholders value NBIC's current products, we have previously reported on the important role that nonfederal partners in the biosurveillance enterprise, particularly because most of the resources necessary to generate biosurveillance information are outside of the federal government.[31] The federal departments and agencies with primary biosurveillance roles, as outlined in this report, have a variety of relationships and agreements with nonfederal partners to facilitate partnership and information sharing. We note that NBIC's authorizing legislation calls for NBIC to work with state and local entities in coordination with, and through when possible, its federal partners and these existing relationships.

Chris Currie
Director, Homeland Security and Justice

APPENDIX I: BIOSURVEILLANCE RESPONSIBILITIES OF THE NATIONAL BIOSURVEILLANCE INTEGRATION SYSTEM PARTNERS

We surveyed and interviewed officials from 19 federal departments and their component agencies across 13 of the 14 departments and agencies that compose the National Biosurveillance Integration System (NBIS).[32] We refer to these 19 agencies as NBIS-partner agencies, and we categorized these into three groups:

- *Primary biosurveillance agencies:* Have major biosurveillance mission responsibilities that include collecting or analyzing biosurveillance information for the purposes of detecting, monitoring, or responding to biological events.
- *Support biosurveillance agencies:* Do not have missions that directly involve disease detection and monitoring; however, they collect data and information or have subject matter expertise that may be useful to efforts to detect, monitor, or respond to biological events.
- *Biosurveillance information consumers:* Generally do not produce information that is useful for biosurveillance, but consume such information because biological events can affect their main mission and they may have a particular role to play in responding to an event.

We developed these categories based on each partner's roles and responsibilities related to biosurveillance. Table 3 includes brief summaries of the NBIS partners, including agency type, mission, domains, and biosurveillance responsibilities.[33]

Table 3. Biosurveillance Responsibilities of the National Biosurveillance Integration System Partners

Agency: Animal and Plant Health Inspection Service (APHIS)	
Department: U.S. Department of Agriculture	
Type of biosurveillance agency: *Primary biosurveillance agency*	Mission: To safeguard the health, welfare and value of American agriculture and natural resources, which includes issues related to animal and plant health, wildlife damage and disease management, regulation of genetically engineered crops and animal welfare and protection of public health and safety as well as natural resources that are vulnerable to invasive pests and pathogens.
Main biosurveillance domains: *Animal health* *Plant health*	Biosurveillance roles and responsibilities: APHIS is responsible for implementing and conducting national measures to detect, control, or eradicate certain livestock and poultry diseases (such as diagnostic testing), as well as safeguard U.S. agriculture and natural resources against the entry, establishment, and spread of economically and environmentally significant pests. APHIS is also responsible for emergency response to an economically devastating or highly contagious animal disease—for example, by determining the veterinary and other expertise needed to respond.
Agency: Armed Forces Health Surveillance Center (AFHSC)	
Department: Department of Defense (DOD)	
Type of biosurveillance agency: *Primary biosurveillance agency*	Mission: To provide timely, relevant, actionable, and comprehensive health surveillance information to promote, maintain, and enhance the health of military and military- associated populations.
Main biosurveillance domains: *Human health*	Biosurveillance roles and responsibilities: AFHSC coordinates surveillance activities by tracking and monitoring the health of the U.S. uniformed services. AFHSC is the central source for DOD-level medical surveillance data, including current and historical data on diseases and medical events (e.g., hospitalizations, laboratory tests, and immunizations) throughout service members' military careers. According to agency officials, AFHSC also monitors the health of military and civilian populations around the world for diseases that could affect the U.S. military.

<table>
<tr><td colspan="2">Agency: Centers for Disease Control and Prevention (CDC)</td></tr>
<tr><td colspan="2">Department: Department of Health and Human Services</td></tr>
<tr><td>Type of biosurveillance agency: Primary biosurveillance agency</td><td>Mission:
To protect America from health, safety, and security threats; fight disease and support communities and citizens to do the same; and increase the health security of the nation.</td></tr>
<tr><td>Main biosurveillance domains:
Human health
Animal health</td><td>Biosurveillance roles and responsibilities:
CDC is the lead federal agency for human health surveillance and develops strategies for conducting surveillance of diseases in humans, including coordinating with other agencies to monitor zoonotic diseases, which can be transferred between animals and humans.</td></tr>
<tr><td colspan="2">Agency: U.S. Customs and Border Protection (CBP)</td></tr>
<tr><td colspan="2">Department: Department of Homeland Security</td></tr>
<tr><td>Type of biosurveillance agency: Primary biosurveillance agency</td><td>Mission:
To safeguard America's borders thereby protecting the public from dangerous people and materials while enhancing the Nation's global economic competitiveness by enabling legitimate trade and travel.</td></tr>
<tr><td>Main biosurveillance domains:
Human health
Animal health
Plant health
Homeland security</td><td>Biosurveillance roles and responsibilities:
CBP provides frontline personnel and assets at ports of entry in both U.S. and foreign ports where CBP performs hands-on inspections to determine that imports are free of pests and humans are free of disease, according to agency officials. CBP interacts with other agencies in this function, for example enforcing Department of Agriculture regulations on plants and animals or referring sick passengers to the Centers for Disease Control and Prevention. CBP also screens for chemical, biological, radiological, nuclear, and explosives, and maintains an ongoing mechanism to assess threats.</td></tr>
<tr><td colspan="2">Department: Department of Energy (DOE)</td></tr>
<tr><td>Type of biosurveillance agency: Biosurveillance information consumer</td><td>Mission:
To ensure America's security and prosperity by addressing its energy, environmental, and nuclear challenges.</td></tr>
<tr><td>Main biosurveillance domains: Human health</td><td>Biosurveillance roles and responsibilities:
According to officials, DOE largely uses biosurveillance information for occupational health reasons. However, DOE's National Laboratories can provide subject matter expertise to biosurveillance partners on an as-needed basis.</td></tr>
</table>

Table 3. (Continued)

Department: Department of State (DOS)	
Type of biosurveillance agency: *Biosurveillance information consumer*	Mission: To shape and sustain a peaceful, prosperous, just, and democratic world and foster conditions for stability and progress for the benefit of the American people and people everywhere.
Main biosurveillance domains: *Human health*	Biosurveillance roles and responsibilities: DOS collects information from its medical units abroad to support its health preparedness and response activities, rather than as an early warning function, according to officials. DOS's Office of International Health and Biodefense focuses on global health security, pandemic preparedness, and emerging issues, such as new outbreaks of disease and how science and technology affect medicine and public health. Agency officials noted that DOS generally plays a policy and facilitation role, not a programmatic role.
Department: Department of Transportation (DOT)	
Type of biosurveillance agency: *Biosurveillance information consumer*	Mission: To ensure a fast, safe, efficient, accessible and convenient transportation system.
Main biosurveillance domains: *Human health*	Biosurveillance roles and responsibilities: DOT is a consumer of biosurveillance information because biological events can affect the national transportation system, according to officials. DOT provides information and guidance to stakeholders—state officials, private industry, transportation workers, and the travelling public—regarding biological events and epidemics. In addition to providing guidance when requested, DOT also has responsibility for ensuring the safe transporting of biohazardous waste and the highest-level biological agents.
Department: Department of Veterans Affairs (VA)	
Type of biosurveillance agency: *Support biosurveillance agency*	Mission: To serve America's Veterans as their principal advocate to ensure that they receive medical care, benefits, social support, and lasting memorials, and to promote the health, welfare, and dignity of all veterans in recognition of their service to this nation.

Department: Department of Veterans Affairs (VA)	
Main biosurveillance domains: *Human health*	Biosurveillance roles and responsibilities: VA patient health data can contribute to biosurveillance efforts, according to officials. In the event of an emergency, VA also can play a role in response by, for example, providing health care to the public through its infrastructure, which includes 167 VA Medical Centers.
Agency: Environmental Protection Agency (EPA)	
Type of biosurveillance agency: *Primary biosurveillance agency*	Mission: To protect human health and the environment. EPA's purpose includes ensuring that all parts of society—communities; individuals; businesses; and state, local and tribal governments—have access to accurate information sufficient to effectively participate in managing human health and environmental risks.
Main biosurveillance domains: *Environmental safety and security*	Biosurveillance roles and responsibilities: EPA is developing guidance materials and training to promote the water sector's adoption of contamination warning systems based on lessons learned from five EPA-funded pilot projects, according to officials. EPA also runs the nationwide RadNet system that monitors the nation's air, precipitation, and drinking water to track radiation in the environment.
Agency: Federal Bureau of Investigation (FBI)	
Department: Department of Justice	
Type of biosurveillance agency: *Support biosurveillance agency*	Mission: To protect and defend the United States against terrorist and foreign intelligence threats; to uphold and enforce the criminal laws of the United States; and to provide leadership and criminal justice services to federal, state, municipal, and international agencies and partners.
Main biosurveillance domains: *Homeland security*	Biosurveillance roles and responsibilities: As a member of the intelligence community, the FBI gathers, shares, and analyzes intelligence information on threats to the United States, including those involving biological agents.
Agency: U.S. Food and Drug Administration (FDA)	
Department: Department of Health and Human Services (HHS)	
Type of biosurveillance agency: *Primary biosurveillance agency*	Mission: To protect public health by ensuring the safety, efficacy, and security of human and veterinary drugs, biological products, medical devices, our nation's food supply, cosmetics, and products that emit radiation.

Table 3. (Continued)

Agency: U.S. Food and Drug Administration (FDA)	
Main biosurveillance domains: *Food safety and defense Human health*	Biosurveillance roles and responsibilities: FDA monitors events related to FDA-regulated products, such as vaccines, medicine, medical devices, food, tobacco products, and animal feed, according to agency officials. FDA's role is to ensure that its regulated products are safe and effective, but also to understand emerging threats that may require FDA to take action. For example, FDA can work with industry partners to increase vaccine production if a particularly virulent strain of influenza begins to spread.
Agency: Food Safety and Inspection Service (FSIS)	
Department: U.S. Department of Agriculture	
Type of biosurveillance agency: *Primary biosurveillance agency*	Mission: To ensure that the nation's commercial supply of meat, poultry, and processed egg products is safe, wholesome, and correctly labeled and packaged.
Main biosurveillance domains: *Food safety and defense Human health*	Biosurveillance roles and responsibilities: In collaboration with federal, state, local and territorial public health officials, FSIS conducts surveillance by monitoring foodborne incidents, initiating foodborne illness investigations, and responding to consumer complaints.
Agency: National Center for Medical Intelligence (NCMI)	
Department: Department of Defense (DOD)	
Type of biosurveillance agency: *Primary biosurveillance agency*	Mission: To lead DOD activity for the production of medical intelligence and prepare and coordinate integrated, all-source intelligence for the DOD, other government agencies, and international organizations on foreign health threats and other medical issues to protect U.S. interests worldwide.
Main biosurveillance domains: *Homeland security*	Biosurveillance roles and responsibilities: As a member of the intelligence community, the Defense Intelligence Agency's NCMI analyzes intelligence to identify biological threats originating from outside the United States for DOD, according to agency officials. The center also assesses the extent to which foreign countries are able to address these threats and the impact that these threats may have on foreign militaries.

Agency: National Oceanic and Atmospheric Administration (NOAA)	
Department: Department of Commerce	
Type of biosurveillance agency: *Support biosurveillance agency*	Mission: To understand and predict changes in climate, weather, oceans, and coasts; share that knowledge and information with others; and conserve and manage coastal and marine ecosystems and resources.
Main biosurveillance domains: *Environmental safety and security*	Biosurveillance roles and responsibilities: NOAA provides information that might be relevant for those involved in monitoring and detecting biological events, such as situational awareness of weather events, according to agency officials. Warm temperatures, drought conditions, hurricane landings, and other weather events monitored by NOAA can influence biological events. For example, NOAA is working with other federal agencies to use NOAA's technical expertise in developing weather forecast models to help other agencies develop models to predict dengue epidemics.
Agency: Office of Emergency Management	
Department: Department of the Interior (DOI)	
Type of biosurveillance agency: *Primary biosurveillance agency*	Mission: To, among other responsibilities, coordinate prevention, planning, response, and recovery programs and policies for all types of hazards and emergencies that affect federal lands, facilities, infrastructure, and resources, as well as Tribal lands and insular areas.
Main biosurveillance domains: *Human health Animal health*	Biosurveillance roles and responsibilities: According to agency officials, DOI's Office of Emergency Management monitors wildlife health through the Fish and Wildlife Service and the National Park Service. The Fish and Wildlife Service performs disease tests of birds and hunter-captured animals in its refuges. The National Park Service monitors the health of human visitors to the national parks as well as wildlife that live in the parks.
Agency: Office of Intelligence and Analysis (I&A)	
Department: Department of Homeland Security (DHS)	
Type of biosurveillance agency: *Support biosurveillance agency*	Mission: To equip federal, state, local, and tribal governments and the private sector with the intelligence and information they need to keep the homeland safe, secure, and resilient.

Table 3. (Continued)

Agency: Office of Intelligence and Analysis (I&A)	
Main biosurveillance domains: *Homeland security*	Biosurveillance roles and responsibilities: As a member of the intelligence community, I&A reviews all source intelligence, including biosurveillance information, to identify threats to the U.S., according to agency officials. I&A analysts look for threats, including terrorist threats aimed at agriculture and chemical, biological, radiological, nuclear, and high explosives threats. I&A develops analysis and information for DHS senior leadership, federal, state, and local government officials, and private stakeholders.
Agency: Office of the Assistant Secretary for Preparedness and Response (ASPR)	
Department: Department of Health and Human Services (HHS)	
Type of biosurveillance agency: *Primary biosurveillance agency*	Mission: To lead the nation in preventing, preparing for, and responding to the adverse health effects of public health emergencies and disasters.
Main biosurveillance domains: *Human health Animal health*	Biosurveillance roles and responsibilities: ASPR tracks public health incidents and all-hazard incidents that potentially affect human health, such as hurricanes, earthquakes, and zoonotic diseases, according to agency officials. HHS collects and integrates such data through an around-the-clock operations center and disseminates this data to stakeholders both inside and outside of HHS. In addition, ASPR maintains the U.S. International Health Regulation's National Focal Point, which coordinates public health information from other countries as well as international organizations like the World Health Organization.
Agency: United States Geological Survey (USGS)	
Department: Department of the Interior	
Type of biosurveillance agency: *Primary biosurveillance agency*	Mission: To provide reliable scientific information to describe and understand the Earth; minimize loss of life and property from natural disasters; manage water, biological, energy, and mineral resources; and enhance and protect quality of life.
Main biosurveillance domains: *Animal health Environmental safety and security*	Biosurveillance roles and responsibilities: USGS maintains the National Wildlife Health Center, which identifies, controls, and prevents wildlife losses from diseases as well as conducts research to understand the impact of diseases on wildlife populations, and devises

Agency: United States Geological Survey (USGS)	
	methods to more effectively manage these disease threats. In addition, USGS monitors the environment. For example, according to agency officials, USGS is currently studying naturally occurring anthrax in top soil and looking at environmental drivers, such as drought, that can expose more topsoil and in turn expose more naturally occurring anthrax spores that can infect both animals and people.
Agency: United States Postal Service (USPS)	
Type of biosurveillance agency: *Support biosurveillance agency*	Mission: To provide prompt, reliable, and efficient postal services to all areas of the nation.
Main biosurveillance domains: *Homeland security*	Biosurveillance roles and responsibilities: USPS screens collection mail using biohazard detection units located in mail-processing plants to detect the presence of anthrax, according to agency officials. The U.S. Postal Inspection Service, a law enforcement agency within USPS, responds to suspicious packages and powders.

Source: GAO structured interviews with NBIS partners GAO analysis of agency documents. | GAO-15-793

APPENDIX II: BIOSURVEILLANCE AGENCIES' SOURCES FOR INFORMATION THAT ENHANCES SITUATIONAL AWARENESS OF BIOLOGICAL EVENTS

We conducted a Web-based survey of the 19 National Biosurveillance Integration System (NBIS) partners to identify the federal agencies from which they obtain information that contributes to their agency's situational awareness of biological events.

Because this was not a sample survey, it has no sampling errors. However, the practical difficulties of conducting any survey can introduce errors, commonly referred to as nonsampling errors. We took steps in developing the questionnaire, collecting the data, and analyzing them to minimize such nonsampling errors. We conducted pretests with 3 agencies to help ensure that the questions were clear and unbiased, and that the questionnaire did not place an undue burden on respondents. An independent reviewer within GAO also reviewed a draft of the questionnaire prior to its administration. We made appropriate revisions to the content and format of the survey questionnaire based on the pretests and independent review. The survey was administered on the Internet from March 25, 2013, to May 15, 2013. To increase the response rate, we followed up with emails and personal phone calls to the experts to encourage participation in our survey. We received responses from all 19 agencies in our population (100 percent response rate). Based on comments we received from two agencies, we also conducted two follow-up phone calls with officials at these agencies who responded to our survey to verify their answers to survey questions about the federal agencies from which their agency obtains information that contributes to their agency's situational awareness of biological events. We made appropriate changes to the responses recorded on these officials' questionnaires to reflect the clarifications made during these phone calls. When we analyzed the data, an independent analyst verified all programs. Because this was a Web-based survey, respondents entered their answers directly into the electronic questionnaire, eliminating the need to key data into a database, minimizing error.

In the survey, we asked each agency whether it obtains information from each of the other agencies in our population, as well as which types of information it obtains from them (perception-, comprehension-, or projection-related information). For the purposes of this report, we use the definition of situational awareness that the *NBIC Strategic Plan* uses in the articulation of its mission. The definition has its basis in the work of Mica Endsley, who described situational awareness as having three elements: (1) perception that a situation has occurred, (2) comprehension of the situation's meaning, and (3) projection of the event's likely course in the near future.[34] We performed a network analysis of these survey data, which is a quantitative and graphical technique for identifying the underlying patterns in a complex system of relationships among entities of interest. Figure 9 illustrates the agency sources from which the primary and support biosurveillance agencies in our survey obtain data that enhances their situational awareness of biological events. For example, officials from the Environmental Protection Agency (EPA) reported that their agency obtains information that enhances all three elements of situational awareness from seven agencies, including the Animal and Plant Health Inspection Service, Centers for Disease Control and Prevention, and National Biosurveillance Integration Center, among others. Further, EPA officials reported that they obtain information that enhances their comprehension and projection of biological events from the Department of the Interior's Office of Emergency Management and the National Center for Medical Intelligence.

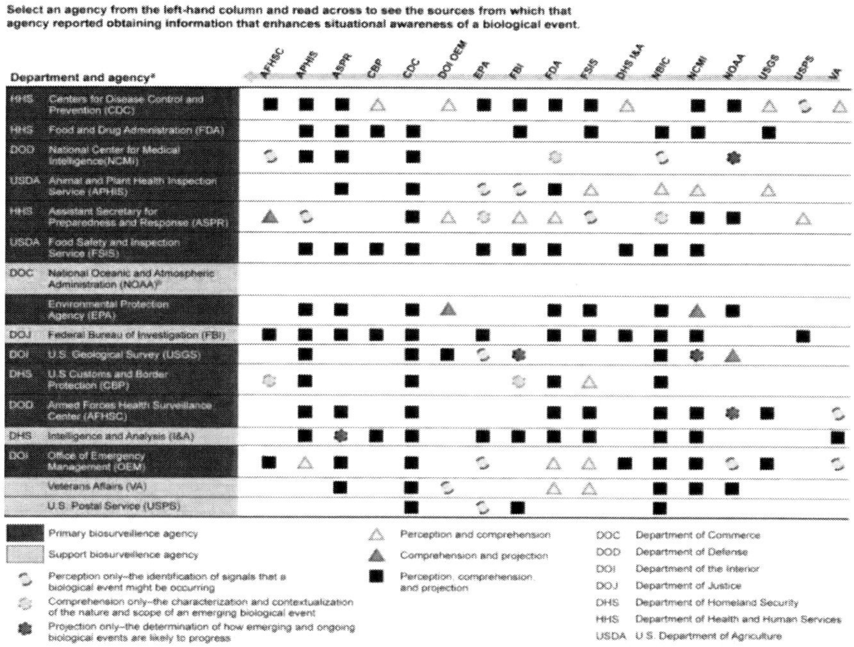

Source: GAO survey of NBIS partners. | GAO-15-793

Notes:

In the online interactive version of figure 9, the size of the circle for an NBIS partner reflects the number of times other NBIS partners identified it as an information source used to enhance situational awareness of a biological event. For the version above in this appendix, NBIS partners are listed down the left-hand column in order of the greatest to the least number of times other NBIS partners identified the agency as an information source that enhances their situational awareness.

[a] Although we obtained information from each NBIS partner identifying the other NBIS partners from which they obtain information that contributes to their situational awareness, we did not collect similar information from NBIC. According to NBIC, the agency relies heavily on products from NBIS partners, such as written reports of partners' analysis of specific events.

[b] We did not collect information from NOAA that identified which NBIS partners that contribute to its situational awareness of a biological event because unlike the other support biosurveillance agencies, officials from NOAA stated that situational awareness and early warning of biological events is of little importance to their agency's primary mission. Officials noted that although their agency can provide information that may be useful to efforts to detect, monitor, or respond to biological events, they maintain situational awareness of biological events only to the extent that it impacts NOAA operations.

Figure 9. Primary and Support Biosurveillance Agencies' Sources for Information that Enhances Situational Awareness.

End Notes

[1] 6 U.S.C. § 195b.

[2] Senior NBIC officials agreed that these three roles are consistent with the center's responsibilities.

[3] For the purposes of this report, we use the definition of situational awareness that the *NBIC Strategic Plan* uses in the articulation of its mission. According to the plan, the definition has its basis in the work of Mica Endsley, a former Chief Scientist of the U.S. Air Force who has written extensively on situational awareness. Endsley described situational awareness as having three elements: (1) perception that a situation has occurred, (2) comprehension of the situation's meaning, and (3) projection of the event's likely course in the near future. Further, the strategic plan notes that shared situational awareness is a common picture or understanding achieved cooperatively by entities that integrate mission essential, overlapping portions of their individual situational awareness for a unified purpose.

[4] GAO, *Biosurveillance: Developing a Collaboration Strategy Is Essential to Fostering Interagency Data and Resource Sharing*, GAO-10-171 (Washington, D.C.: Dec. 18, 2009).

[5] We identify these agencies and describe their biosurveillance responsibilities later in this report, as well as in Appendix I.

[6] Our list initially included 25 agencies, but we later removed 6 of these agencies because we learned that the agency had relatively little direct interaction with NBIC, among other reasons. For example, we initially identified DOI's Fish and Wildlife Service and National Park Service as potential NBIS partners. However, according to DOI officials, these agencies have relatively little direct interaction with NBIC because DOI's Office of Emergency Management, which we did interview, collects information from both agencies and filters it to NBIC.

[7] The Advisory Board serves as the assistant secretary–level body for coordination and communication regarding integrated biosurveillance among NBIC's federal partners. The NBIC Interagency Working Group is to provide support and respond to taskings from the Advisory Board to assist in addressing NBIC operational, programmatic, and scientific issues.

[8] Our survey data were processed into a matrix form readable in the UCINet network analysis package and transformed into a prototype graphic using a set of automated and manual techniques. This prototype was then refined using graphical software such as Adobe Illustrator.

[9] See U.S. Department of Homeland Security, *National Biosurveillance Integration Center Strategic Plan*, Washington, D.C.: Aug. 2012; White House, *National Strategy on Biosurveillance*, Washington, D.C.: July 31, 2012; and Executive Office of the President, National Science and Technology Council, *National Biosurveillance Science and Technology Roadmap,* Washington, D.C.: June 14, 2013.

[10] The *NBIC Strategic Plan* specifically identifies the human, animal, plant, food, and environmental domains. However, because the 9/11 Commission Act states that NBIC is to receive and consider other relevant homeland security information, we also include homeland security as one of the domains. The Homeland Security Act of 2002, defines homeland security information as any information possessed by a federal, state, or local agency that—(a) relates to the threat of terrorist activity; (b) relates to the ability to prevent, interdict, or disrupt terrorist activity; (c) would improve the identification or investigation of a suspected terrorist or terrorist organization; or (d) would improve the response to a terrorist act. 6 U.S.C. §§ 195b(j)(3), 482(f)(1).

[11] Per the 9/11 Commission Act, the term "biological event of national concern" means an act of terrorism involving a biological agent or toxin, or a naturally occurring outbreak of an infectious disease that may result in a national epidemic.

[12] According to the board's charter, the Advisory Board replaced the NBIS Interagency Oversight Council in November 2013 and expanded NBIC's governance to the broader federal biosurveillance community.

[13] Although not within the scope of this review, the national biosurveillance capability also depends upon participation from state, local, and tribal governments, as few of the resources required to support the capability are wholly owned by the federal government. The responsibility and capacity for collecting most information related to plant, animal and human health, food, and environmental monitoring resides within state, local, and tribal governments, or private sector entities—such as hospitals and other private health care providers. For more information on nonfederal biosurveillance, see GAO, *Biosurveillance: Nonfederal Capabilities Should Be Considered in Creating a National Biosurveillance Strategy,* GAO-12-55 (Washington, D.C.: Oct. 31, 2011).

[14] The 9/11 Commission Act does not specify any member agency that must participate in the NBIS, but defines a member agency as any federal department or agency that has entered a memorandum of understanding regarding participation in NBIC. 6 U.S.C. § 195b(j)(4). Seven of the 14 federal partners have or had memorandums of understanding or interagency agreements with NBIC or DHS's Office of Health Affairs as of July 2015. These agreements are generally for the provision of specific personnel or technology, or participation in a joint project.

[15] Although ODNI is represented on the NBIC Advisory Board, officials from NBIC, ODNI, and the Department of Homeland Security's Office of Intelligence and Analysis (I&A) noted that NBIC's relationship with the intelligence community is currently conducted through I&A. According to NBIC officials, the center's relationship with ODNI is new and they have not yet established direct relationships with ODNI. Therefore, we did not include ODNI among the NBIS partners we interviewed and surveyed.

[16] NBIC decommissioned its Biosurveillance Common Operating Network, an open-source search engine, in November 2013, an action that officials stated allowed NBIC to invest in more cost-effective technology. Officials stated that, as an interim measure, this system was replaced by acquiring access to other biosurveillance information feeds from other federal agencies, such as Arkham, and commercial sources. NBIC officials further added that the center is investing in additional capabilities to replace and improve upon the Biosurveillance Common Operating Network capabilities.

[17] Generally, these 5 NBIS partners stated that they did not have a basis to judge because they are biosurveillance information consumers or they considered their role in biosurveillance to be relatively small.

[18] Specifically, these partners reported that they share raw structured data with NBIC through approved channels. Raw structured data include data that have been collected in an electronic format that can be automatically processed by a computer but have not been analyzed to reach conclusions about their meaning, such as whether the data are signs of a potentially catastrophic infectious disease outbreak. All 5 of the NBIS partners that reported sharing such data with NBIC are primary biosurveillance agencies.

[19] 5 U.S.C. § 552a; 552.

[20] See Pub. L. No. 104-191, Title II, Subtitle F, 110 Stat. 1936, 2021 (Aug. 21, 1996) (codified at 42 U.S.C. §§ 1320d–1320d-9); 45 C.F.R. Parts 160, 164.

[21] GAO-10-171.

[22] These thresholds are (1) any indications of biological events manifesting anomalous levels of death, illness, disease, or injury that surpasses agency specific thresholds for information sharing with NBIS; (2) any credible indication of an accidental or intentional misuse of any chemical, radiological, or biological agent that may adversely affect human, animal, or plant health or harm the food supply; (3) any non-routine request for assistance or information from one NBIS partner to another regarding a biological event that may have significance to the larger NBIS community; and (4) any biological event that could reasonably be assessed as being a "high visibility" event requiring awareness of senior leadership.

[23] The agencies and departments represented in the Biosurveillance Indications and Warnings Analytic Community include APHIS, CDC, Department of State, DHS, DOD, HHS's Office of the Assistant Secretary for Preparedness and Response, and the intelligence community.

[24] NBIC officials stated that the BATR is currently being restructured, but did not know when the National Security Council had intended to finalize it.

[25] Out of 13 DHS component databases, the study identified 2 CBP systems as the most useful to NBIC. The Automated Targeting System is an enforcement and decision support system that compares passenger and cargo manifest information against intelligence and other law enforcement data. TECS (not an acronym) is an automated enforcement and antiterrorism database maintained by CBP that provides information for law enforcement and border security purposes.

[26] Officials reported that this includes funds from reprogramming, recessions, and transfers.

[27] GAO-10-171.

[28] Specifically, we found that 12 of the 14 NBIS partners we interviewed at that time expressed uncertainty about the value of participating in the NBIS or confusion about the purpose of NBIC's mission. For more on the agencies we interviewed for that report, see GAO-10-171.

[29] In our structured interviews, we did not specifically ask a question on the extent to which NBIC had improved its products, outreach, coordination, and other activities over time, so it is possible that officials from the other NBIS partners may have also agreed with this statement.

[30] Of the 13 NBIS partners that stated that the concept is very or moderately important, 7 were primary biosurveillance agencies, 4 were support biosurveillance agencies, and 2 were biosurveillance information consumers.

[31] See GAO *Biosurveillance: Nonfederal Capabilities Should Be Considered in Creating a National Biosurveillance Strategy*; GAO-12-55 (Washington, D.C.: Oct 31, 2011).

[32] The Office of the Director of National Intelligence (ODNI) is represented on the National Biosurveillance Integration Center (NBIC) Advisory Board, and is therefore considered by NBIC to be a member agency of the NBIS. However, officials from NBIC, ODNI, and the Department of Homeland Security's Office of Intelligence and Analysis (I&A) noted that NBIC's relationship with the intelligence community is currently conducted through I&A. According to NBIC officials, the center's relationship with ODNI is new and they have not yet established direct relationships with ODNI. Therefore, we did not include ODNI among the NBIS partners we interviewed and surveyed.

[33] The *NBIC Strategic Plan* specifically identifies the human, animal, plant, food, and environmental domains. However, because the 9/11 Commission Act states that NBIC is to receive and consider other relevant homeland security information, we also include homeland security as one of the domains. The Homeland Security Act of 2002, defines homeland security information as any information possessed by a federal, state, or local agency that—(a) relates to the threat of terrorist activity; (b) relates to the ability to prevent, interdict, or disrupt terrorist activity; (c) would improve the identification or investigation of a suspected terrorist or terrorist organization; or (d) would improve the response to a terrorist act. 6 U.S.C. §§ 195b(j)(3), 482(f)(1).

[34] The definition has its basis in the work of Mica Endsley, a former Chief Scientist of the U.S. Air Force who has written extensively on situational awareness. For example, see Mica Endsley, "Toward a Theory of Situational Awareness in Dynamic Systems," Human Factors: The Journal of the Human Factors and Ergonomics Society, (vol. 37, no. 1) 1995; and Mica Endsley and Debra G. Jones, *Designing for Situation Awareness: An Approach to User-Centered Design*. 2nd ed., (Boca Raton, FL) CRC Press, 2011.

In: The National Biosurveillance Integration ... ISBN: 978-1-63484-924-1
Editor: Natasha Jennings

Chapter 2

NATIONAL BIOSURVEILLANCE INTEGRATION CENTER STRATEGIC PLAN*

Department of Homeland Security

EXECUTIVE SUMMARY

The 2010 Department of Homeland Security (DHS) Quadrennial Homeland Security Review states "ultimately Homeland Security is about effectively managing risks to the Nation's security." With risk defined as the likelihood and consequences of potential unwanted events, managing risks from naturally-occurring, accidental, or deliberate biological events such as emerging infectious disease or bioterrorism is difficult to accomplish through activities that attempt to reduce these events' likelihood of occurrence. Although much is being done to prevent these types of events, such events could and do still occur. Instead, activities that mitigate these risks largely focus on reducing, managing, or limiting the consequences of biological events[1] once they begin to occur. Surveillance plays an import role in early detection of such events, allowing an early response, limiting the spread and effects of such events. Doing this effectively requires the earliest possible warning that an event is occurring, as well as continuing shared situational awareness throughout the event, to enable effective decision making regarding what actions should be taken.

---

* This is an edited, reformatted and augmented version of a document issued by the U.S. Department of Homeland Security, November 2012.

The mission of the National Biosurveillance Integration Center (NBIC) is fundamentally about the integration of biosurveillance information to enable early warning and shared situational awareness,[2] and disseminate it to the appropriate people in a timely fashion. The *National Biosurveillance Integration Center Strategic Plan* first provides an overview of national biosurveillance in general, as well as current NBIC activities and operations, then outlines the goals and objectives required to achieve the NBIC's mission over the next five years. These strategic goals, objectives, and activities represent a balance of efforts that enable early warning and shared situational awareness through information ingestion and analysis; synthesis of existing government, private non-governmental, open-source, and classified information; and innovating advanced analytics and models, all in collaboration with federal partners and state, local, territorial, tribal, private, and international stakeholders. NBIC's goals and objectives outlined in this plan include these stakeholders and will be measured for success against specific milestones developed in collaboration with them.

National Biosurveillance Integration Center

Mission: Enable early warning and shared situational awareness of acute biological events and support better decisions through rapid identification, characterization, localization, and tracking.

Strategic Vision: Advance the safety, security, and resilience of the Nation by leading an integrated biosurveillance effort that facilitates early warning and situational awareness of biological events.

The development of this Strategic Plan is the result of a deliberative process examining current capabilities and capability gaps of NBIC and has been created in coordination with NBIC's interagency partners.

This Strategic Plan was developed during a critical time as events[3] with implications for biosurveillance continue to threaten the nation and the world. These events are a reminder that a rigorous national biosurveillance capability is critical to enable early awareness of threats to the nation's health security and, ultimately, to save lives. These ongoing challenges signal the acute need to mitigate the impacts of intentional attacks, natural disease outbreaks, and other biological events through improved information sharing and coordinated analysis.

The *National Biosurveillance Integration Center Strategic Plan* presents a new approach to fully realize the vision of NBIC and articulates goals and objectives to fulfill its vital integration role in the national biosurveillance mission. Following extensive discussions within the federal government and with external groups, this Strategic Plan explains the approach, why it is needed, and how it seeks to achieve the mission of the NBIC and execute the vision of integrating national biosurveillance information through the National Biosurveillance Integration System (NBIS) interagency collaboration, all for the purposes of supporting better-informed decision making.

Four core disciplines have been identified as essential to the biosurveillance integration mission.[4] This Strategic Plan outlines these core disciplines as: 1) collaboration, in which governance improvements and new communication processes and policies will be pursued; 2) information integration and sharing, in which appropriate information technology (IT) systems, business rules, and partner data management/ownership verification will be a priority; 3) analysis, which requires multidisciplinary, cross-cutting, and in-depth analytic support to provide timely and relevant information to support decisions; and 4) user-defined reporting, recognizing that all aspects of NBIC's analysis and products must be tailored and customer-focused. To transform NBIC and continue to mature national capability, these core disciplines will be achieved through accomplishing NBIC's strategic goals and objectives.

Goals for a Successful Center

The strategic goals and objectives outlined in this plan are oriented around the four core disciplines:

1. **Interagency collaboration through NBIS.** As the operational entity for the NBIS, the NBIC must work more closely and effectively with interagency, state, local, territorial, tribal, and private sector stakeholders. Through the management and use of working groups, joint concept of operations (CONOPS) development, provision of technical assistance and integration infrastructures, and other collaborative tools and approaches, the NBIC will both benefit from, and contribute to, the missions of its NBIS partners.

   Development of an NBIC CONOPS through collaboration and coordination with NBIS partners is a top priority for NBIC and will be initiated immediately upon formalization of the Strategic Plan. The NBIC CONOPS will layout the organizational structure of NBIC and

NBIS and describe the specific roles and responsibilities of NBIS partners and stakeholders as they relate to NBIC. The NBIC CONOPS will also clearly define the operational objectives and provide specific operational details of the NBIS biosurveillance process.

2. **Information integration and analysis**. Consolidating information from NBIS partner surveillance systems, enhancing information gap coverage through the addition of stakeholder information, and conducting tailored, direct analysis using appropriate tools and technologies to identify and characterize biological events of national concern will make the NBIC's decision support products more relevant and useful for customers and decision makers.
3. **Effective dissemination of information.** While improved information integration and sound analysis will produce improved decision support products, effective dissemination of those products to the appropriate people in a timely fashion is equally important. Improving real time communication methods with NBIS partners and enhancing intelligence community information sharing will improve the NBIC's ability to effectively inform partners and stakeholders.
4. **Mature and strengthen the Center.** To effectively accomplish NBIC's mission through its strategic goals requires the recruitment, development, and retention of a world-class, multi-disciplinary analytic staff. In addition, NBIC must continue to work with its stakeholders to innovate new ways of leveraging existing data and models, as well as applying advanced analytics to more effectively discern early warning and awareness from available information.

Implementing the Vision

In charting the way forward, this Strategic Plan articulates an "emergent strategy" approach that allows for a series of initiatives that can be measured and validated. Specifically, strategic objectives and activities will be tested with key NBIS partners through small-scale pilot projects to develop building blocks for the operational activities of the NBIC prior to adoption. As outlined in this plan, these pilot projects, as well as other activities, will allow for greater participation at the state and local level, in the private sector, and among non-governmental organizations. Such an approach is prudent as changes in technology, the threat picture, or even in policy or governmental priorities may emerge and affect the strategy during its implementation.

Implementation will be coordinated with the NBIS partners and build from the concepts, measures, and milestones outlined in this document to mature NBIC collaboration, analysis, and operations going forward.

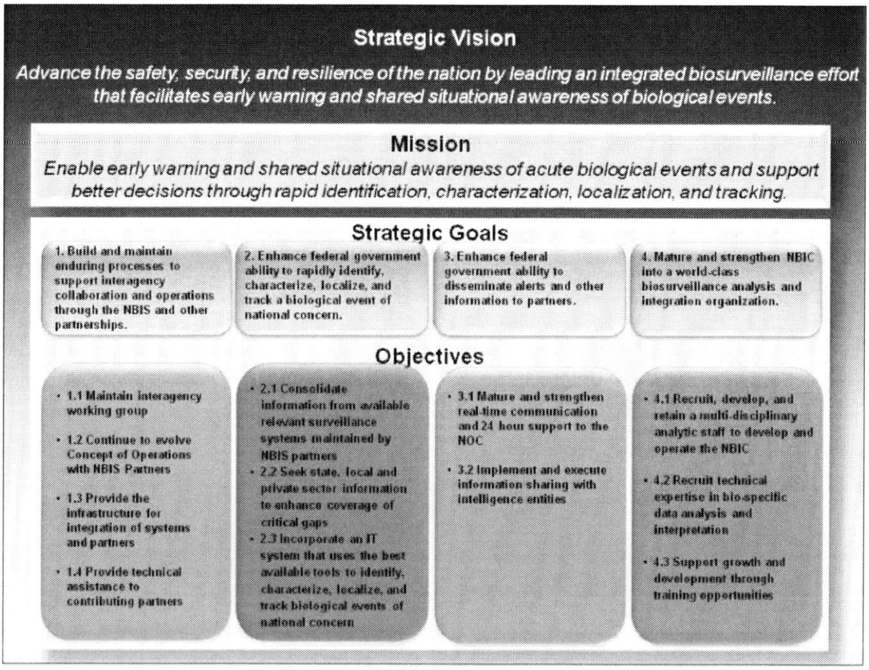

Conclusion

Effective management of risks from biological threats and evolving events depends on early warning and shared situational awareness so that risk management decisions surrounding response and recovery are well-informed. To that end, the federal government performs biosurveillance through several domains: human, animal, plant, food, and environmental health. NBIS member agencies have roles and responsibilities related to each of the domains and NBIC is in a unique position to support those roles and responsibilities and work collaboratively to ensure that health surveillance information in all these domains is analyzed, integrated, shared, and used to make sound risk management decisions that save lives, mitigate socioeconomic impacts, and reduce the likelihood of future reoccurring events. Most of this information does not reside within the federal government but with many biosurveillance stakeholders including state, local, territorial, and tribal (SLTT) governments, the private sector, and the international entities. There is still much to be learned from combining these different information sources.

Having a strong, state-of-the-art NBIC will support these efforts on behalf of, and in collaboration with, the biosurveillance community. This Strategic Plan articulates strategic goals, objectives, and activities essential to achieving its mission. Through the NBIC, and working together with our NBIS partners, we will advance the safety, security, and resilience of the Nation through biosurveillance collaboration, analysis, and integration.

PURPOSE OF THE STRATEGIC PLAN

The *National Biosurveillance Integration Center Strategic Plan* presents a new approach to realizing the vision of NBIC. This Plan identifies core disciplines of biosurveillance integration and addresses the requirement for NBIC to define its goals and objectives necessary to fulfill its vital role in the national biosurveillance mission. This plan is grounded in legislative and presidential direction and is informed by extensive discussions, workshops, and symposiums with the biosurveillance community. As the first Strategic Plan since the establishment of NBIC, this plan explains the approach, why it is needed, and how it seeks to execute the vision of integrating national biosurveillance information.

In implementing this Strategy, some of the aforementioned assumptions and new applications will be tested with key NBIS partners through small-scale pilot projects to develop building blocks prior to adoption by NBIC. A key aspect of the implementation is integrating lessons learned from others in information sharing and best practices into the design of communication tools for stakeholders. To date, a preponderance of efforts has focused at the federal and international level, but there are recognized contributions and strengths at the state and local level, as well as private sector. For all activities outlined in the "Path toward Implementation" section, attention will be focused on the capabilities and enhancements available through strong input and integration of this information and ensuring the mutual exchange for the decision support and full situation awareness. A transformed NBIC will require flexibility, implementation of bold new approaches, and requirements that will encourage buy-in and support of the users with increased emphasis on the state and local stakeholders. When achieved, this Strategy describes a NBIC that will support each partner's mission and provide valuable and accessible information for decision making.

This document was written in coordination with the NBIS partners and is outlined in three sections. The first section describes the state of biosurveillance to include the role of the NBIC and the NBIS partners in national biosurveillance integration. The second describes the current state of NBIC and its capabilities and activities to date. Lastly, the third section outlines the goals, strategic objectives, and activities necessary to build on the current capabilities, address the challenges, and implement a path towards making success for NBIC a reality. The third section identifies new processes, products, and enabling technologies with measures and milestones for each of the activities.

PART I: STATE OF BIOSURVEILLANCE

A. Background

In 2004, the President tasked[5] the Department of Homeland Security (DHS) to develop a national biosurveillance integration system in coordination with appropriate federal departments and agencies for rapid recognition and warning of an intentional dispersal of biological agents. At the time, the nation's capability to detect biological attacks was dispersed across federal departments and agencies, each with its own mission, function, and corresponding perspective. Members of the biosurveillance community envisioned a center where information from across multiple domains and fields, from both governmental and non-governmental sources, would be integrated and analyzed. It was believed that key analysts would be able to coordinate and integrate streams of biosurveillance information rapidly and take critical, life-saving actions promptly. Although these capabilities remain dispersed across the departments and agencies, the solution is in leveraging those capabilities to enhance our ability to share and integrate the dispersed information. This vision is similar to that in the law enforcement and intelligence communities that have increased focus on information sharing and integration since the attacks of September 11, 2001.

> ***Biosurveillance*** is the science and practice of managing human, animal, plant, food, and environmental health-related data and information for early warning of threats and hazards, early detection of events, and rapid characterization of the event so that effective actions can be taken to mitigate adverse health, social, and economic effects.*
>
> * Derived from biosurveillance definition in February 2010 National Biosurveillance Strategy for Human Health to include all biosurveillance domains.

A number of policies and directives have highlighted biosurveillance as a critical capability to the United States biodefense efforts and the importance of integrating the biosurveillance information at the federal level and, in some instances, with state and local entities. In 2004, the President issued two directives, Homeland Security Presidential Directives (HSPD) 9 and 10. Specifically, HSPD-9 directs various departments and agencies to develop surveillance systems as appropriate to the mission and domain focus of that agency and provides a reminder that biosurveillance includes more than the traditional human health information but also information from the food and agricultural sector. HSPD-10 identifies biosurveillance as a pillar of biodefense and directs Homeland Security, in coordination with the appropriate federal departments and agencies, to integrate these biosurveillance efforts. As the conversation on national biosurveillance coalesced, a program to address the need for coordination and integration was transferred from the DHS Office of Infrastructure Protection to the Office of the Chief Medical Officer in 2006. Also in 2006, the Pandemic All Hazards Preparedness Act required the U.S. Department of Health and Human Services (HHS) to develop and sustain essential public health security capabilities, including disease detection and investigation. HSPD–21, *Public Health and Medical Preparedness*, builds upon principles set forth in HSPD– 10, explicitly defines biosurveillance, and provides a detailed explanation of what a nationwide, robust, and integrated biosurveillance capability must include (e.g., epidemiological surveillance) and accomplish.

When Congress passed the Implementing Recommendations of the 9/11 Commission Act of 2007 (Public Law 110-53), one of the key provisions was to codify the federal government's expectations for biosurveillance integration and coordination. The law directed the Secretary of Homeland Security to "establish, operate, and maintain a National Biosurveillance Integration Center (NBIC)" having a mission to (1) "enhance the capability of the federal government to rapidly identify, characterize, localize, and track a biological event of national concern[6] and disseminate alerts and other information to Member Agencies and, in coordination with them to agencies of state, local, and tribal governments" and, (2) "oversee the development and operation of the National Biosurveillance Integration System (NBIS)."

National Biosurveillance Integration Center Mission, as Codified in Public Law 110-53

Codified in Sec 1101 of P.L. 110-53, the law directed the Secretary of Homeland Security to "establish, operate, and maintain a National Biosurveillance Integration Center (NBIC)" having a mission to (1) "enhance the capability of the Federal Government to rapidly identify, characterize, localize, and track a biological event of national concern and disseminate alerts and other information to Member Agencies and, in coordination with them to agencies of State, local, and tribal governments to enhance the ability of such agencies to respond to a biological event of national concern" and, (2) "oversee the development and operation of the National Biosurveillance Integration System (NBIS)."

Additional Presidential Directives, legislation, and department and agency strategies continue to shape the federal government's biosurveillance efforts. These include, but are not limited to, HHS' 2009 *National Health Security Strategy* and the 2010 *National Biosurveillance Strategy for Human Health.* In 2010, the Secretary of DHS established the first Quadrennial Homeland Security Review to outline the strategic framework to guide the activities of participants in homeland security toward a common end. The review calls out the need to focus on maturing and strengthening the homeland security enterprise and aligns well with NBIC's focus on enhancing a broad national culture of cooperation to "prevent and protect against terrorism" and "ensuring resilience to disasters", two key missions of the homeland security enterprise. In 2011, the Food and Drug Administration (FDA) Food Safety Modernization Act specifically directs the HHS Secretary, through the Director of the Centers for Disease Control and Prevention (CDC), to enhance foodborne illness surveillance systems by "integrating foodborne illness surveillance systems and data with other biosurveillance and public health situational awareness capabilities at the federal, state, and local levels, including by sharing foodborne illness surveillance data with the National Biosurveillance

Integration Center; and other activities as determined appropriate by the Secretary.[7]" This further highlights the necessity for information integration and sharing across multiple domains to provide improved broad situational awareness potential biological events.

In 2011, the President issued the *Presidential Policy Directive (PPD) 8: National Preparedness* with the goal of strengthening the security and resilience of the United States through systematic preparation for the threats that pose the greatest risk to the security of the Nation. As deliverables from PPD-8, the National Preparedness Goal and National Planning Frameworks highlight the importance of biosurveillance, integration, and information sharing within the Protection mission area.[8] Most recently, the President released the *National Strategy for Biosurveillance* which sets forth the United States Government approach to strengthen our national biosurveillance enterprise and describes a core set of functions critical to the National Strategy's success. The NBIC Strategic Plan is aligned with the National Strategy's concepts and approaches and rooted in the same goal to provide critical information and ongoing situational awareness that enables better decision making.[9]

B. Establishing a Common Understanding

As Congressionally directed, NBIC resides within the DHS Office of Health Affairs (OHA) to coordinate the comprehensive integration of national biosurveillance to better inform homeland security situational awareness. NBIC is the coordinating group responsible for supporting the NBIS partners and establishing a capability to integrate information across the public and private domains. Such coordination requires the collaboration of stakeholders with differing missions, organizational cultures, and nomenclature to effectively support the response to events using near real time information gathered from multiple sources, analyzed by experts, and presented in usable formats across the NBIS to the nation's decision makers.

NBIC, largely through interactions with the NBIS partners, collaborates with the interagency community to acquire, integrate, analyze, and disseminate information pertaining to emerging biological events and their impact on U.S. interests.

National Biosurveillance Integration System Mission

The National Biosurveillance Integration System (NBIS) enhances the identification, location and tracking of biological events potentially impacting homeland security by uniquely integrating information and leveraging interagency communications and relationships. NBIS supports prevention and mitigation of such events by providing timely notifications and ongoing situational awareness to enhance response of government agencies. (Established by the NBIS partners and effective June 30, 2010)

The NBIS is a consortium of federal partners that was established to rapidly identify and monitor biological events of national concern. NBIS collaborates among federal partners and state stakeholders to collect, analyze, and share human, animal, plant, food, and environmental biosurveillance information with the NBIC. As described in the P.L. 110-53 in 2007, NBIS was originally intended to be an information technology (IT) system that enabled integration of numerous complex, structured and unstructured data relevant to biosurveillance. However, since 2007, it is clear that comprehensive data sources as envisioned in P.L. 110-53 either do not exist or are subject to a variety of information sharing challenges that make a large IT-centered solution less feasible than originally imagined. However, NBIC does currently field a limited IT system, the Biosurveillance Common Operating Network (BCON), which collects and shares open source information in support of its mission. NBIC and its partners now describe NBIS in terms of the biosurveillance community of federal partners as opposed to an IT system. In 2010, the NBIS partners established a formal mission statement to solidify their role with regards to NBIC.

I. Understanding Integration and Shared Situational Awareness as an Unique Role of the Center

The goal of an integrated biosurveillance effort across public and private sectors is hindered by the lack of a standard scope for biosurveillance. Before significant progress is made, a common understanding of terms used between public and private biosurveillance entities must be achieved. HSPD-21 defines *biosurveillance* as "the process of active data-gathering with appropriate analysis and interpretation of biosphere data[10] that might relate to disease activity and threats to human or animal health – whether infectious, toxic, metabolic, or otherwise, and regardless of intentional or natural origin – in order to achieve early warning of health threats, early detection of health events, and overall situational awareness of disease activity."[11] NBIC proposes to incorporate the HSPD-21 concepts and adapt and expand the HHS definition of biosurveillance put forth in the 2010 *National Biosurveillance Strategy for Human Health* to reflect the cross-domain nature of biosurveillance and its ability to inform mitigation efforts beyond health effects. ***Biosurveillance** is the science and practice of managing human, animal, plant, food, and environmental health-related data and information for early warning of threats, early detection of events, and rapid characterization of events so that effective actions can be taken to mitigate adverse health, social, and economic effects*. NBIC is foremost an integrator of biosurveillance information as it relates to information shared through a collaborative process where information exchange agreements have been developed and are followed. NBIS partners integrate data within their biosurveillance domain, and share this information with NBIC after being analyzed by their subject matter experts.

Given the importance of integration in NBIC's mission and activities, providing a working definition of what that means is important. Information integration is the combining of information from different sources and providing partners and stakeholders with a synthesized, unified view of the information, and what it could mean. Information integration has a greater impact than information aggregation alone, which is just the collecting of information to give users a single place of access. Integration takes this a step further by providing a broad perspective of the impact of the combined whole of aggregated information.

Consequently, NBIC is more than a repository for reports from itself and other NBIS partners. Although this is a useful function, NBIC (in full collaboration with its partners) connects, correlates, and contextualizes (not just aggregates) information through the production and dissemination of its analytic products. Done well, integration requires constant information updates, strong collaborative relationships, and strong analytic expertise. NBIC's integrating role enhances the federal government's ability to provide early warning and shared situational awareness beyond information aggregation.

Situational awareness is broadly defined as the perception of elements in the environment within a given time and space, the comprehension of their meaning, and the projection of their status in the near future.[12] As highlighted in HSPD-21, biosurveillance, at a national level, is an important part of the process for achieving shared situational awareness of the biological event of national concern. ***Shared situational awareness*** *is best understood as a common picture or understanding achieved cooperatively by entities that integrate mission-essential, overlapping portions of their individual situational awareness for a unified purpose.*[13] In the context of this document, shared situational awareness is established through the integration and sharing of biosurveillance information, and is part of the larger situational awareness established by the National Operations Center (NOC) Common Operating Picture (COP).

> ***Situational awareness*** is the perception of elements in the environment within a given time and space, the comprehension of their meaning, and the projection of their status in the near future.*
>
> * Mica Endsley, Toward a theory of situation awareness in dynamic systems (Human Factors, 1995b

Emerging events require a set of high-consequence decisions be made based upon preliminary, incomplete, and often inconclusive information across multiple domains including human, animal, plant, food and environmental. Each department and agency (federal, state, and local) has a primary mission, often focused on a single domain, and subsequently a set of decisions and actions that must be made in a shared risk environment. Shared situational awareness of the broader biological domain established from integrating information across the individual missions may provide insights that cannot be gleaned in isolation. The shared analysis may enhance the likelihood of identifying an event earlier and with more certainty. Going forward, NBIC will remain the integrator of national biosurveillance information by fostering an improved environment for shared situational awareness and decision support within the biosurveillance sphere.

C. Core Disciplines of Integrated Biosurveillance

This Strategic Plan is the result of a deliberative process examining current capabilities and capability gaps of NBIC and has been created in coordination with the NBIS partners and other key stakeholders. Based on these efforts, this plan outlines four core disciplines that have been identified as essential to the biosurveillance integration mission.[14] These core disciplines, which include collaboration, information integration and sharing, analysis, and user-defined reporting are critical to successful biosurveillance and reflected in the Strategic Goals and Objectives discussed in detail in Part III: Path toward Implementation.

Collaboration

Open and mutual communication, cooperation, and trust is necessary for successful information sharing among NBIS partners.[15] NBIC must leverage the expertise of its NBIS partners and establish processes that provide access to timely information and the appropriate personnel from these partner agencies. Clarity on agency roles and responsibilities as relevant to their relationship with NBIC will improve issues of overlapping agency authorities for integration. Overall, NBIC must foster a trusted information sharing environment that encourages members in the biosurveillance community to share and discuss information so incidents can be identified and assessed earlier.

In order to implement improvements to NBIC, OHA and the NBIS partners will be fully engaged in the planning, development, and deployment activities of NBIC. Particularly important to the ongoing success of national biosurveillance integration is the governance of the biosurveillance community. The NBIS partners have expressed that a shared, participatory governance model is desired. Governance will be important to address early on to ensure full participation and build trust with the stakeholders in order to implement a successful NBIC.[16] As noted in detail in Strategic Objective 1.2, an NBIC CONOPS will be created through a collaborative interagency process. The CONOPS will address roles and responsibilities of the NBIC in conjunction with stakeholders, including customers, distribution of products, and the process for sharing information both pre- and post- event identification (before and after resources and capabilities outlined in the National Response Framework (NRF) are activated). The CONOPS will define procedures for aggregating, integrating, and analyzing biosurveillance data both pre- and post- event, and will also address and clarify the role of the NBIC regarding other standing protocols.

Information Integration and Sharing

Information integration and sharing are integral components to developing improved individual situational awareness and shared awareness among partnering organizations.[17] Establishing information needs and information sharing agreements driven by the information owner and determining the value proposition for the NBIS partners are essential for success of NBIC. As necessary, NBIC will adopt IT platforms designed to accept information from different platforms and provide ways to integrate that information. This will enable consistent and timely information sharing that can be leveraged by NBIS partners with minimal capability or the infrastructure to support a biosurveillance system. In collaboration with the lead federal partners, NBIC will support the broadly recognized need to develop a federal registry of information sources, systems, or programs to lay the foundation for sharing.[18]

Analysis

A fully effective biosurveillance system is not only dependent on the clear delineation of information requirements and appropriate information sources but also on the robust analytic schema and expertise essential to support the discovery of emerging threats. Taking advantage of the current efforts in new analytic tools and processes within the research community and surveillance daily operations, as well as new computing technologies, will help build more efficient and customer-defined decision support. These user-defined responsive tools will enable analysts to more easily conduct analysis but do not replace their essential expertise in this process. Multidisciplinary, cross-cutting, and in-depth analytical support within NBIC and across agencies is necessary to provide real time and ongoing analyses to provide timely, relevant information supporting decisions of senior leaders.[19] Examination and testing of these analytic and computing tools in real time biosurveillance activities with networked subject matter expert analysts is a high priority milestone for a successful NBIC.

User-Defined Reporting

With the final value and outcome of an efficient NBIC focused on providing subject matter expert (SME) analysts and leaders at all levels with the best consolidated information for decision making, it must first be determined what information the NBIS partners need and what they can provide among the NBIS partners. Those needs will be compared to the senior leaders needs, and the NBIS will collectively determine solutions for how to best provide the requested information in multiple formats for a diverse audience of end users. Currently, NBIC ingests a large quantity of open source information on any health event, however minor or significant, in any geographic location. Reporting should integrate and analyze the vast open source information and provide usable insights of incidents that might not be seen in isolation. NBIC must continue to improve its reporting and tailor its products to provide decision making support for SME analysts, senior leadership, and policymakers. NBIC must identify who the "customer" of information integration is – the targeted leadership within agencies, outside agencies, and in state, local, territorial, and tribal (SLTT) governments.

NBIC reports should include where possible, analysis of linkages, causality, trends, and information visualization to guide decision making. Many information sharing experts have addressed interfaces, graphs, visual analytics, mapping and other information sharing mechanisms that will be explored in order to best communicate NBIC analyses.

PART II: THE NATIONAL BIOSURVEILLANCE INTEGRATION CENTER DAILY OPERATIONS

A. Current Operations Overview

In its national biosurveillance role, the NBIC functions as an integration center. Memoranda of understanding (MOU), interagency agreements, and standard operating procedures have shaped how the NBIC conducts daily biosurveillance integration. As part of NBIC's emerging strategy approach, the interaction with its stakeholders will continue to influence the evolution of NBIC daily operations. The following overview captures how NBIC operates today.

A Day in the Life at the Center

Continuous biosurveillance monitoring activities produce the baseline that permits NBIS partners, including NBIC, to provide indications and warnings. This results in a shared situational awareness and subsequently assists forecasting of future disease incidence, impact, and necessary mitigation measures by NBIS partners. Through collaboration, information integration and sharing, and analysis, NBIC provides stakeholder-defined biosurveillance reporting. This section will focus solely on the current, daily NBIC operations that include both steady state continuous open source biosurveillance and near real time biosurveillance decision support capabilities.

B. Continuous Biosurveillance: A Daily NBIS Collaboration

NBIC performs continuous open source biosurveillance while simultaneously collaborating with its NBIS partners. These partners provide subject matter expertise that NBIC uses in its daily operations, the integration of national biosurveillance information.

I. Daily Analytic Production Process

Surveillance begins each weekday morning by reviewing information and data collected since the previous review. Information regarding disease outbreaks and biological events of concern or interest is collected manually 24 hours a day by NBIC analysts and OHA Watch Officers in the NOC. Potentially relevant information is also collected through the use of the Biosurveillance Common Operating Network (BCON), an automated information gathering tool that ingests data from tens of thousands of information feeds. Information collected by BCON includes such varied sources as open source media, information aggregation and dissemination systems (such as ProMed and OIE – World Organization for Animal Health), NBIS partner input, individual internet searches, and specialized portals.

NBIS Partners

- Department of State
- Department of Justice
- Department of Interior
- Department of Commerce
- Department of Agriculture
- Department of Defense*
- Department of Health and Human Services
- Department of Transportation
- Department of Veterans Affairs
- Department of Homeland Security*
- Environmental Protection Agency
- U.S. Postal Service

*DOD and DHS are two of the 17 member agencies of the Intelligence Community

The overall process described above relies heavily on analyst experience and subject matter expertise, as well as voluntary interagency collaboration. For this expertise, the NBIC has two sources that allow collaboration with subject matter expertise from lead agencies to inform national biosurveillance integration. The first is the aforementioned broader NBIS community that includes the other federal partners, plus state and local government stakeholders. In addition, the NBIC can access OHA expertise residing outside the NBIC.

II. Biodefense - NBIC Relationship within OHA and the NOC

OHA leads DHS' biodefense activities[20], to include responsibilities outlined in the HSPD-10, *Biodefense for the 21st Century,* consistent with formal DHS planning processes, end-to-end planning for biological attacks, biosurveillance integration, operational early warning systems, and veterinary, food and agro-defense.

The NBIC partners with OHA's BioWatch, Chemical Defense Program, and the Food, Agriculture, and Veterinary Defense (FAVD) branches. These partnerships allow NBIC to leverage in-house expertise and advance information sharing through these OHA programs with additional federal and SLTT stakeholders.

Under the Office of Operations Coordination and Planning, the NOC is the primary national-level hub for all domestic situational awareness and incident response coordination. In addition to the OHA programs previously mentioned, OHA maintains constant staffing of the OHA Watch Desk within the NOC to serve as a conduit for information exchange between OHA, DHS components, and the interagency. NBIC information sharing is coordinated with the OHA Watch Desk and routine biosurveillance reporting is shared with the NOC. Some NBIS partners also maintain a physical presence at watch desks within the NOC.

During routine operations within the NOC, NBIC analysts perform the majority of routine staff work involved in biosurveillance integration through direct interaction via phone calls and emails with designated peers in other government agencies during normal working hours. At all hours, the Public Health Service officers staffing the OHA Watch Desk perform associated biosurveillance functions in coordination with NBIC personnel and personnel from the partner agencies working within the NOC. As these interactions are currently dependent upon the specific partners involved and the information sought, a detailed CONOPS for NBIC interaction with NBIS partners through the NOC is needed and proposed in this document (see Strategic Objective 1.2). Some partners prefer direct analyst-to-analyst communication to perform staff work as efficiently as possible during routine operations and request the use of the NOC's formal operations center-to-operations center request for information (RFI) process be limited to significant events or unusual requests. Other partners prefer that all communication be routed and logged through the formal NOC RFI process.

During the initial stages of a potentially significant biological event, the NBIS Protocol may be activated, which generates an interagency teleconference to communicate and gather biosurveillance-related information among federal agencies when a situation meets one or more of the established threshold criteria. If there are any indications of a nefarious or potential intentional event, NBIC will immediately notify the FBI.

When the appropriate senior leadership does decide that a biological event has risen to a level of concern sufficient to form a Crisis Action Team (CAT) within the National Operations Center (NOC), interagency information exchange is then coordinated through the NOC CAT in accordance with established procedures. The NBIC ceases formal, direct interagency information coordination for the event and functions as a member of the CAT through the designated representative(s) (see Strategic Objective 3.1).

C. Real Time Biosurveillance Decision Support Capabilities

The other element of the NBIC's daily biosurveillance effort is to provide decision making support in as near to real time as attainable. Continuous biosurveillance forms the baseline that allows recognition of indicators that an event may be developing or is crossing a threshold to becoming a biological event of national concern. Since continuous biosurveillance is ongoing across all NBIS partners, the NBIC is positioned as a hub for information sharing. The NBIC's ability to integrate and analyze information and communicate effectively the shared awareness of a situation enables leaders to make better-informed decisions, even in the face of incomplete or constantly changing information.

I. Rapid Turnaround Analyses

A major value of the NBIC is its ability to provide analysis in near real time for questions posed by the NBIS partners, DHS leadership, and state and local government officials. The NBIC is frequently charged with providing short turnaround, expert responses to requests from senior federal leadership. NBIC SMEs, using available expertise and resources, collaborate with SMEs from NBIS partner agencies to provide the most complete response possible given the time frame. Examples of products delivered include such items as subject-specific papers, verbal briefings, expert opinions or perspectives, and document reviews.

II. Information Sharing for Decision Support

NBIC prepares and distributes reports for a variety of audiences. These reports include:

- Federal Biosurveillance Common Operating Picture (BCOP) Reports: subject-specific reports available to more than 500 users from multiple federal agencies via the NBIC Homeland Security Information Network (HSIN) portal.
- SLTT BCOP Reports: Biosurveillance reports made available to SLTT stakeholders via the Minerva HSIN, Health Security Intelligence Enterprise HSIN, and BioWatch portals.
- Reporting and Monitoring List: daily synopsis of the most critical issues being tracked by the NBIC as well as other items of interest such as recently posted BCOP reports. The product is distributed by the OHA Watch Desk at the NOC to more than 500 federal government officials and redistributed by the DHS Office of Operations Coordination & Planning to a broader distribution list of federal officials.
- NBIC General Disease Infodoc: a group of documents and reports with corresponding links identified by NBIC analysts as having relevance to the NBIS mission based on interagency-developed Critical Information Requirements (CIRs). It is distributed daily and with the agenda prior to the weekly federal interagency call. The analysts generate the Infodoc using BCON.
- HSIN Operational Analytic Exchange: Permits secure but informal correspondence and collaboration regarding raw information for NBIS member collaboration in an unclassified environment.

III. Personnel Support to DHS Crisis Response Teams

NBIC has periodically provided analyst/SME personnel to temporary support teams formed by DHS to respond to potential crisis events. These crisis response teams form the DHS component of the interagency response efforts. Past examples include the 2009 H1N1 outbreak and the 2010 Deepwater Horizon oil spill.

IV. NBIS Protocol Activation

An important aspect of NBIC's information sharing and coordination role is its ability to activate the NBIS Protocol to include alerting the NBIS partner agencies and generating Spot Reports.

NBIS Protocol

The NBIS Protocol is a mechanism to bring federal NBIS partners together on a short-notice teleconference to share information on a potentially significant biological event. It can be initiated at the request of any NBIS partner and is an example of a unique capability of the NBIC that helps enable national biosurveillance integration. The Protocol is activated when a situation meets one or more of the threshold criteria and is requested by a NBIS agency. It will be used as outlined in the decision tree below.

Value Added

NBIS Protocol activations demonstrate the ability of the NBIC to rapidly bring together subject matter experts across the federal government representing the human, animal, plant, food, and environmental domains. The purpose of the Protocol activation is to ensure information is shared across the NBIS and assess that information in order to characterize an unfolding event and provide early warning in the case of a potential biological event of national concern. The NBIS Protocol provides a forum for timely national biosurveillance integration that enables information sharing early in a biological event's discovery and development phase to facilitate information analysis and provide reports for decision makers. Ultimately, this early decision making support helps to mitigate the impact that the biological event could have on the nation to include decreasing the time of response as well as decreasing the overall duration and severity of a biological event. By quickly bringing together the whole of the federal biosurveillance enterprise, the Protocol enhances the goal of timely and integrated national biosurveillance.

NBIS Protocol Flow Chart

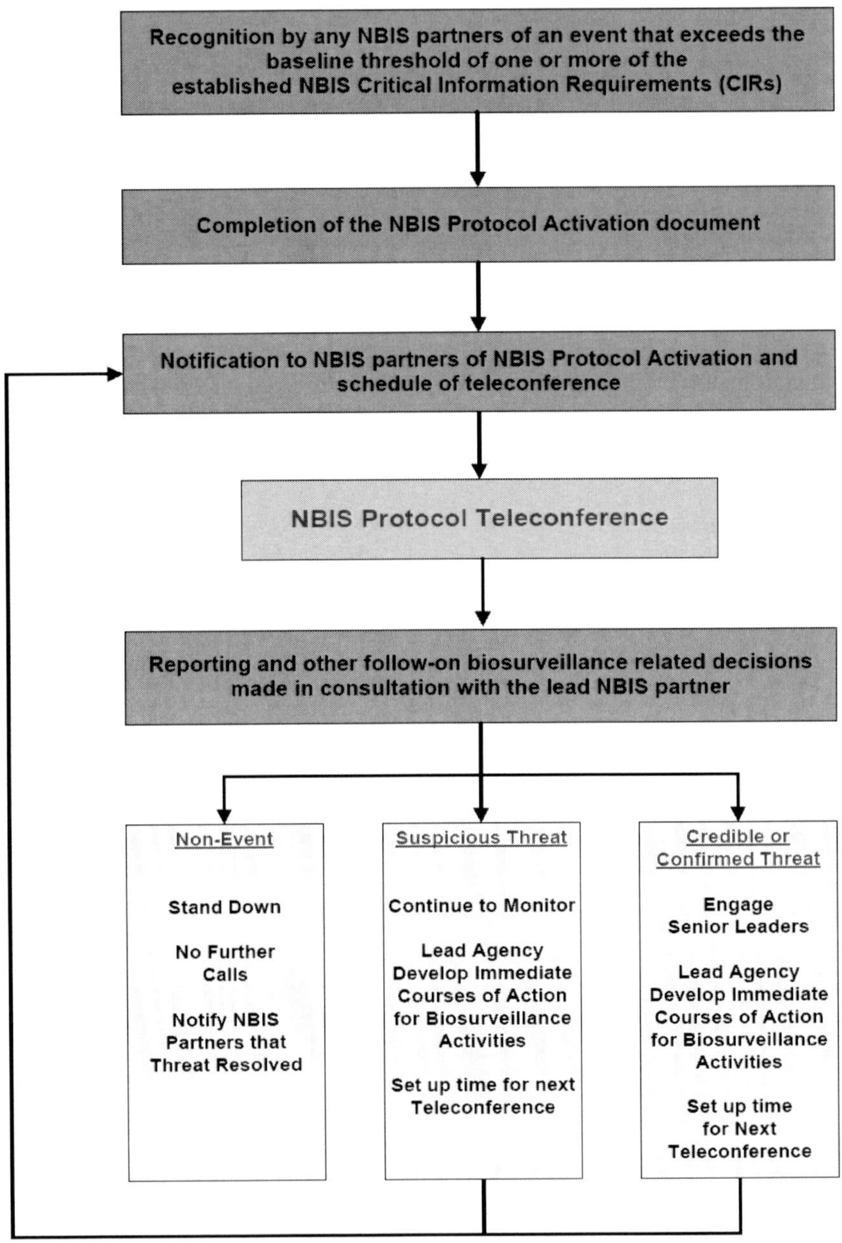

PART III: THE PATH TOWARD IMPLEMENTATION (FY14 – FY18) A. STRATEGIC GOALS AND OBJECTIVES

NBIC Strategic Vision: Advance the safety, security, and resilience of the Nation by leading an integrated biosurveillance effort that facilitates early warning and shared situational awareness of biological events.

NBIC Mission: Enable early warning and shared situational awareness of acute biological events and support better decisions through rapid identification, characterization, localization, and tracking.

According to the 2010 DHS Quadrennial Homeland Security Review, "ultimately Homeland Security is about effectively managing risks to the Nation's security."[21] With risk defined as the likelihood and consequences of potential unwanted events,[22] managing risks from man-made or naturally-occurring biological events such as bioterrorism or emerging infectious disease is difficult to accomplish through activities that attempt to reduce an event's likelihood of occurrence. Instead, activities that mitigate these risks largely focus on reducing, managing, or limiting the consequences of biological events once they begin to occur. To do this effectively requires advanced warning that an event is occurring, combined with continued situational awareness throughout the event to enable effective decision-making with regards to what management actions should be taken.

The mission of the NBIC is fundamentally about enabling early warning capabilities alongside continued situational awareness and disseminating information to the right authorities in a timely fashion. As described in detail in this section, NBIC Strategic Goals, Objectives, and Activities represent a balance of efforts that produce early warning and situational awareness through information ingestion and analysis, synthesis of existing government and open-source information, and innovation of advanced analytics and models; all in collaboration with federal, SLTT, private, and international sectors. The NBIC Goals and Objectives outlined below intersect these sectors with milestones to measure their success.

The development of the *National Biosurveillance Integration Center Strategic Plan* provides planning guidance for both near term and FY14 - FY18 budget direction. The five-year plan will be updated annually. The publication of this plan within FY12 is the result of a process examining current capabilities and capability gaps of NBIC in collaboration with NBIS stakeholders.

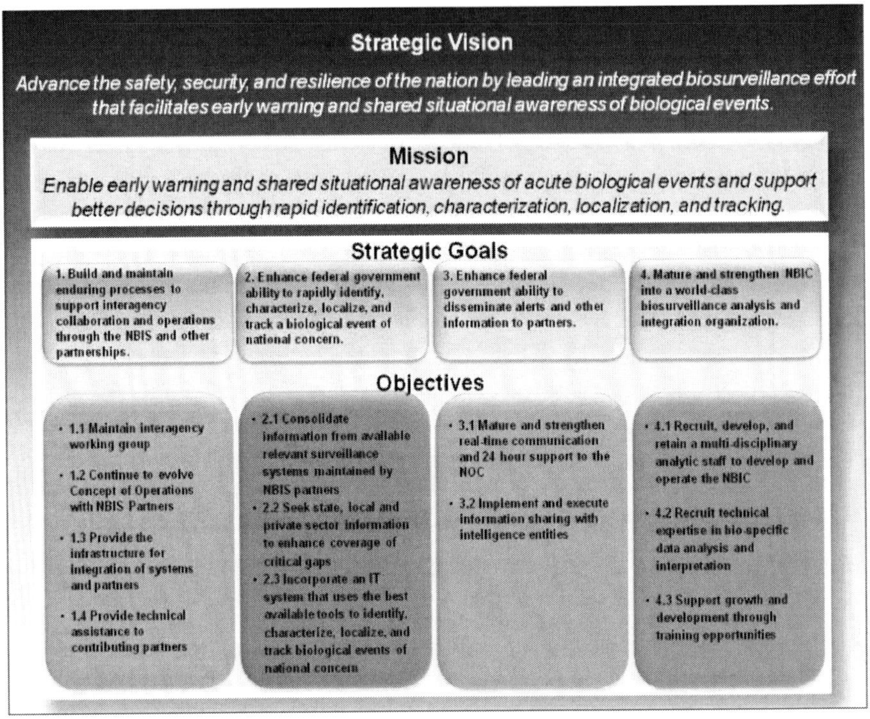

B. An Emergent Strategic Plan: Vision for the Next Five Years

This plan was developed through a deliberative process that includes views from biosurveillance stakeholders as well as the informed inputs of outside studies. This is an emergent strategic plan that began with the NBIC's initial operational capability in September 2008 and reflects the collective experience of a body of partners and stakeholders both inside and outside of NBIS. A previous model does not exist. This plan provides direction to OHA and the NBIC and will be revised periodically as the biosurveillance community and requirements evolve. This direction reflects the maturing and strengthening of NBIC in its integration role in national biosurveillance.

OHA and NBIC have been conducting an analysis of NBIC capability gaps. Filling these gaps will enhance capabilities in collaboration, information integration and sharing, analysis, and user-defined reporting and integration. These challenges will be overcome by a combination of policy, mitigation strategies, and funding solutions. This plan identifies specific programmatic milestones required to accomplish NBIC's mission.

While this implementation plan targets the five year period from FY14 to FY18, OHA has undertaken several initiatives in the near term to respond to identified capabilities gaps. Some of these initiatives are in the form of pilot programs, which focus around specific scenarios across the food, agriculture, and human health/emerging disease events and also on functional areas such as state and local integration, usage of social media, and advanced analytics. These initiatives will focus on making unique contributions to NBIS by advancing the collective knowledge in various, unexplored topic areas to develop and validate new tools for use across the NBIS that fill current gaps and minimize duplication of efforts across NBIS partner activities. NBIS partners will provide input into the pilots and metrics for success. The five year implementation plan including the FY12 – FY13 near–term initiatives and pilot programs are outlined below.

The following strategic goals and objectives are derived from the Congress-defined NBIC mission in P.L. 110-53. Each goal incorporates the core disciplines of collaboration, information integration and sharing, analysis, and user-defined reporting to different degrees depending on the goal.

Strategic Goal 1:

Build and maintain enduring processes to support interagency collaboration and operations through the NBIS and other partnerships.

As a core discipline, collaboration with our partners and stakeholders is essential for successfully achieving national biosurveillance integration. Collaboration is through both the NBIS and the broader biosurveillance community. NBIC must work closely and effectively with federal, SLTT, and private sector entities. The following objectives and activities will guide and support the NBIC in accomplishing this goal.

Strategic Objective 1.1

Maintain an interagency group to facilitate interagency cooperation and to advise the Director of the NBIC regarding recommendations to enhance the biosurveillance capabilities of DHS and the NBIS.

Activity 1.1.1: Revised NBIC Governance Model

NBIC will adopt a model of governance that provides for both centralized and distributed responsibilities, recognizing the importance of considering input from key stakeholders.[23] Within this model, a new NBIC Advisory Board will be created to review, consult, and provide feedback about enterprise strategies and information management policies (e.g., establishing a hierarchy of business rules for use of analyzed sources, determining defensibility of input information, establishing a biosurveillance lexicon), setting of priorities as well as performance metrics of the enterprise and the system to monitor and evaluate the effectiveness of collaboration.[24] The Advisory Board replaces the NBIS Interagency Oversight Council (NIOC) in order to expand responsibilities and involvement in governance to the broader federal biosurveillance community. Participation will go beyond the existing federal NBIS partners with a goal of being more inclusive than the current model. It will include the White House National Security Staff (NSS) and key partners across the federal interagency with biosurveillance mission areas essential for shared situational awareness, potentially including the representatives of the Sub-Interagency Policy Committee for Biosurveillance and the current NIOC representatives. The Board will be implemented in FY12, with initial convening in early FY13.

One of the first tasks of the Advisory Board will be to identify functions that would be the primary responsibility for implementation (e.g., information management responsibilities common to the entire system, establishing architecture and technology standards, and operation of an integration center/network security) by the operating entity, the NBIC. With consideration that it would be impractical for the senior level leadership comprising the NBIC Advisory Board to complete all of these tasks, the existing NBIS Interagency Working Group (NIWG) will assist as requested by the Advisory Board members.

The Advisory Board will initially be convened by the NSS. Once all members have fully agreed to a governance structure, the NSS will transition its role as convener of the Advisory Board to OHA. The Board will then decide upon a co-chair to serve with the OHA Assistant Secretary[25] who will rotate among the Board members to ensure that different agency needs are represented and the enterprise has a shared understanding of the issues to inform operations and evaluate success. The Advisory Board can also establish working groups as needed or as requested by the members for certain operational issues. These working groups could be assigned a specific task, or set up for specific event activities, depending on the needs of the Advisory Board. The current NIWG will remain a permanent working group to support the general working level tasks for the NBIC activities of the Advisory Board. Moving forward, the Board and working group functions may evolve to meet the needs of the NBIS partners.

Initiated in FY13 and finalized in FY14, the Advisory Board will oversee the formulation of a communication plan to better engage SLTT and international stakeholders through associations and professional organizations representing the domains monitored by the NBIC. Stakeholder engagement will also be coordinated with the designated sector-specific agency for any engagement with SLTT entities or the private sector. These stakeholders will provide critical feedback and identify needs and gaps to the NBIC and Advisory Board on issues related to biosurveillance policies and practices. As appropriate, the NBIS partners who have authorized and established relationships will leverage subject matter experts across the biosphere to address operational and information sharing aspects related to special interest topics or events.

Activity 1.1.2: Operations Development Team

The Operations Development Team will support the maturation and strengthening of NBIC operations through analysis, research, and outreach to meet stakeholders' expectations. Operations Development is not research and development but the interface with biosurveillance innovation opportunities. Operations Development will interact in three domains: federal/state programs, public/private sector programs, and broader science interface. The team will be responsible for engagement with the various public and private sector programs, specifically for executing the incorporation of new capabilities into NBIC, including those identified during various pilot programs. Moreover, OHA will establish a Science Advisory Group to inform the Operations Development Team integration effort. This group will consist of members from the OHA medical staff, DHS Science and Technology (S&T), National Biosurveillance Advisory Subcommittee, the White House Office of Science and Technology's Biosurveillance S&T Working Group, and NIWG recommended representatives. As appropriate, other entities, such as the Institute of Medicine, could be invited to participate.

The NBIC, supported by the Operational Development Team, will organize, based on the recommendations from the Advisory Board, an annual Industry Day/Stakeholder Workshop in FY13. The goal of the Industry Day/Stakeholder Workshop will be to bring together experts and stakeholders across the federal government and private sector to discuss critical issues surrounding national biosurveillance integration, best practices used in public and private entities, and new technologies to inform technology and information management strategies to address those issues to enhance efficiency and effectiveness of the NBIC. This will provide a unique opportunity for industry representatives to showcase their capabilities and ensure NBIS partners are apprised of innovative technologies that can enhance the integrated biosurveillance system and the products and activities of the NBIC.

In addition to the Industry Day/Stakeholder Workshop, the Operational Development Team will be dedicated to working with NBIS partners to identify operational development objectives and maintain involvement throughout the requirements generating process to ensure capabilities are developed based on user needs. This group will be informed by the NBIC Advisory Board.

Activity 1.1.3: Establish a Lessons Learned Registry of Major National Biosurveillance Efforts

The NBIC will maintain a lessons learned library of after action reports that follow major national biosurveillance events. The types of after action reports will be based on recommendations of NBIS partners. Reports will normally be recommended by NBIS partners for such events as NBIS Protocol activations or efforts made by NBIS partners following major events (e.g., 2010 Deepwater Horizon oil spill, 2011 Japanese earthquake and tsunami, 2011 Clenbuterol in China, 2011 *E. coli* in Europe). The NBIC will collect after action reports that are authored by either the NBIC or NBIS partners.

Strategic Objective 1.2

Continue to evolve and complete the NBIC CONOPS with the NBIS partners following completion of the NBIC Strategic Plan.

Activity 1.2.1: Clarify Roles and Responsibilities among the NBIS Partners

Because of differing perceptions of roles and responsibilities among the NBIS partners and the SLTT, international and private sector stakeholders, it is essential to work together to further delineate and agree on respective roles and responsibilities. Agreement on the respective roles and responsibilities will be accomplished in FY13.

This strategy is part of the OHA effort to define the NBIC's future strategic direction. Just as a strategic plan is necessary to affect NBIC's mission as mandated by Congress, so is a CONOPS necessary to define how the NBIC works daily within DHS and with its NBIS partners. In FY13 - 14, the NBIC will establish a working group and develop, in collaboration with its NBIS partners, a CONOPS that defines specific formal processes through which the NBIC executes its mission and interacts with partners. This process will be informed by the NBIC Advisory Board and its working groups, as well as the emerging strategy that will be formed at the national level through the NSS. Specifically, the CONOPS interagency working group and subsequently developed document will address the following items:

- engagement with various partners and stakeholders (e.g., DHS Sec, NSS, NBIS partners, NOC, etc.);
- products required by various partners and stakeholders and the appropriate timing of sharing data/information;
- aggregation, integration, and analysis of biosurveillance information prior to a biological incident and in the early stages of characterizing a biological incident pre-activation of resources and capabilities as outlined in the NRF and during a biological incident when NRF mechanisms are activated;
- process for external entities sharing of information with NBIC (via conference calls, reporting, situation reports, etc) post activation of NRF mechanisms;
- identify NBIC's role in response/recovery operations or supporting the NOC once a biological incident is known;
- ensuring NBIC protocols for biological incidents are consistent, to the extent possible, with protocols for other incidents involving other hazards;
- integration of NBIC indications and warnings and alert and notification protocols through the NOC are fully integrated into their normal and bio reporting systems/procedures;
- codification of NBIC's existing integrated process for indications and warnings and alert and notification protocols with FEMA procedures for alert and notification;
- determining the appropriate synchronization and integration of various interagency biological protocols.

Strategic Objective 1.3

Provide the infrastructure for integration, including information technology systems and space, and support for personnel from NBIS partners with sufficient expertise to enable analysis and interpretation of information.

Activity 1.3.1: Liaison Officer Infrastructure Support

The NBIC currently has one on-site liaison officer (LNO) from the USDA FSIS and is in final discussions about bringing in another LNO from the Department of Veterans Affairs in 2012. NBIC provides the work space, information technology support, and access to both classified and unclassified systems. The NBIC will continue to support current and future LNOs with the appropriate infrastructure to ensure adequate interagency collaboration whether their presence is physical or virtual, part-time or full-time.

Strategic Objective 1.4

Provide technical assistance, as appropriate, to all federal, state, local, and tribal government entities and private sector entities that contribute information relevant to the operation of the NBIC.

Activity 1.4.1: Technical Assistance to Biosurveillance Sectors

Public Law 110-53 directs the NBIC to provide technical assistance to the various sectors where the NBIC conducts biosurveillance. Below are examples of such technical assistance. While the NBIC is charged to disseminate alerts and other information to SLTT governments, it fully coordinates this information sharing with and through federal departments and agencies when working with SLTT stakeholders. Existing relationships between federal partners and SLTT stakeholders provide communications channels within the NBIS; the following information integration and sharing efforts are meant to enhance and leverage existing federal–state relationships and not to create redundant channels.

BCON RSS Feeds

Tailored Really Simple Syndication (RSS) feeds to NBIS partners based on user-specified keywords, topics, and taxonomies within BCON will target the right information to the right organizations. As an example, NBIC is providing RSS feeds containing BCON data to the National Collaborative for Bio-Preparedness (NCB-Prepared), an important pilot project in North Carolina evaluating the use of new data sources, analytic approaches, and mechanisms for collaboration for biosurveillance. The RSS feeds include open source biosurveillance data from North Carolina and its four neighboring states that they do not already have readily compiled and organized. This activity is developing a methodology whereby states can have access to BCON RSS feeds. The goal is to be able to provide these feeds to all 50 states and four territories by the end of FY14.

BCON-X

BCON-X is the transition of the BCON tool to the DHS Cloud environment. This will manage costs and provide scalable capabilities and capacity as have been previously described. In addition, this additional functionality will provide external stakeholders with greater access to the BCON tool, which the NBIS member agencies have requested. This effort is dependent on the outcome of the BCON assessment currently underway but is poised to occur in FY13/14.

Engagement through Minerva

A. State and local. The NBIC will deploy the SLTT BCOP, called "Minerva", to all 50 states. The NBIC launched a pilot program to four states, Minnesota, New Jersey, North Carolina, and Washington, in late 2010 to provide state and local governments with a BCOP accessible through a HSIN portal. As of April 2012, 50 states and the District of Columbia have access to this system.

In FY13, NBIC will seek funding to provide for the required specialized technical support to integrate the growing state outreach with Minerva BCOP.

B. Territorial and tribal. In FY13, OHA seeks to expand and complete Minerva deployment to territorial and tribal entities.

International Engagement

NBIC will partner with the Department of State to develop a CONOPS for sharing information with Canadian and Mexican authorities through FY13. These activities will greatly expand NBIC's situational awareness with international stakeholders whose proximity to the United States could provide early warning of events.

A. Canada. In FY12, the NBIC will initiate increased information sharing with Canada. Their advanced market economy and shared interests with the United States offer a natural open space for mutual biosurveillance information sharing.

B. Mexico. Through OHA, the NBIC will initiate contact with Mexican government health authorities. As one of the only two nations contiguous to the United States, many nationals from each country cross the U.S.-Mexico border routinely creating a means of rapid disease transmission. Sharing of biosurveillance information would be mutually beneficial to the two countries.

OHA will seek to leverage existing federal government efforts taken under the Beyond the Borders initiative and the North American Plan for Animal and Pandemic Influenza.

Strategic Goal 2:

Enhance federal government ability to rapidly identify, characterize, localize, and track a biological event of national concern by integrating and analyzing information relating to human health, animal, plant, food, and environmental monitoring systems (both national and international).

Integration and analysis of shared information allows NBIC to build the baseline understanding and general situational awareness. This steady-state, baseline surveillance is critical to allow recognition of the occurrence of a biological event and also when it crosses a threshold in becoming a biological event of national concern. The integration and analysis of information also supports forecasting potential impacts to assist with informing mitigation efforts. The core disciplines of information integration and sharing and analysis will be accomplished through the following objectives and activities.

Strategic Objective 2.1

Consolidate information from relevant and available surveillance systems maintained by NBIS partners to detect biological events of national concern across human, animal, and plant species.

Activity 2.1.1: DHS Data Integration

One of the unique aspects of DHS compared to other agencies with a role in biosurveillance is its large and highly-distributed operational workforce. Recognizing that many of these operational personnel are located in areas of interest for biosurveillance (ports, borders, and airports, among others), DHS operational Components present a largely untapped potential resource for early warning. Accordingly, the Office of Management and Budget recommended that OHA and the broader DHS review internal DHS Component data sources that would be beneficial for inclusion into NBIC data sharing pilots.

In response to this request, OHA has conducted a Departmental data call in collaboration with the DHS Office of the Chief Information Officer (OCIO) to identify information sources that capture or could support biosurveillance. These efforts will increase the information sharing landscape of NBIC and establish improved information access to relevant, authoritative, and trusted data within DHS. Providing access to secure DHS data that can be trusted will improve the data quality and confidence level of NBIS information. NBIC expects to initiate potential data migration/integration agreements with DHS Components in FY12 and to have integrated one or more DHS biosurveillance data systems by the end of FY13. The meta-data regarding biosurveillance systems, programs, and tools defined by the CDC-led Federal Biosurveillance

Working Group will be collected as part of this integration process as needed for a federal cross-agency registry effort.

Activity 2.1.2: Scenario-Based Pilot Programs

In FY12 – FY13, NBIC will engage with its initial set of pilot projects to test and evaluate common information sharing processes and platforms and diverse analytic approaches to determine the best information-sharing structure that is needed for NBIC going forward. Although the exact scope and nature of the individual projects remain in the planning and development stage, it is envisioned that several fast-track initiatives will be conducted with those parties already working closely with the NBIS partners. These initiatives will focus on making unique contributions to the NBIS by advancing the collective knowledge in various unexplored topic areas. It will be designed to develop and validate new tools that fill current gaps while avoiding duplication of NBIS partner activities.

The NBIS partners are currently reviewing the proposed scenario-based pilot projects and are encouraged to provide additional suggestions for pilots in order to identify areas of greatest significance to the NBIS partners. NBIC has proposed pilots across the broad sectors of food, agricultural, and human health/emerging disease surveillance.

Several basic principles will drive the development and evaluation of these pilots:

- Leverage current existing assets for an efficient, scalable, useable, and cost effective structure;
- Apply new and existing successful analytic structures and tools for integration and user adoption;
- Create an open, supported, information-sharing, and problem solving environment to promote partner experimentation and collaboration;
- Define measures and benchmarks for success and design a strategy to incorporate measurable integrated information sharing criteria;
- Examine and clarify underlying assumptions for successful integration parameters and components; and
- Measure and validate results after a defined period to determine success for a larger implementation of the process, tool, or policy.

The criteria for selecting the pilot programs relate to the core disciplines of NBIC but focus on how the program could benefit the larger NBIS community:

Collaboration

- Does the NBIS partner(s) consider it "their pilot"?
- Does this pilot bring in a new partner?
- Were the metrics jointly defined?
- Is the partner part of the evaluation process?

Information Sharing and Integration

- Does this bring together three or more information sets?
- Will this information provide added value to the NOC and support informed decision making?

Analysis

- Can the tool be leveraged beyond the purpose of the individual pilot?

User-Defined Reporting

- Can reports be tailored to different end-user groups?

Activity 2.1.3. Information Sharing Agreements (ISAs)

NBIC will develop an Information Sharing Agreement in collaboration with the NBIS agencies. The USDA FSIS began negotiating an ISA with NBIC in FY12. The objective is to complete this series of agreements by the end of FY14.

Strategic Objective 2.2

Seek state and local biosurveillance information as well as private sources of surveillance information both foreign and domestic, when such sources would enhance coverage of critical surveillance gaps.

Activity 2.2.1. Function-Based Pilot Program: National Collaborative for BioPreparedness (NCB-Prepared)

The NCB-Prepared is a public-private partnership to develop, test, and implement an advanced biosurveillance system beginning in North Carolina. It is a collaborative effort of academic, government, and industry leaders focused on developing a local, bottom-up approach to public health and emergency medical responsiveness and awareness. The NCB-Prepared is creating a comprehensive statewide biosurveillance system for analyzing data from a variety of health, food, social, environmental, and animal sources to provide early outbreak detection and situational awareness of health events. The strategy calls for the continued use of this program as one of its function-based pilot programs for not only state/local engagement but also for private sector engagement, with the goal of evaluating approaches and data sources for scalability to the national level.

This system is innovative in three ways: 1) it gathers and analyzes early biological event information that other current surveillance systems do not use, such as Emergency Medical Services and Poison Control Center data, 2) applies advanced analytics to that data, eventually to include predictive forecasting and optimization, improving the knowledge that can be derived from available data, and 3) develops new approaches to collaboration with state and local entities and data owners.

In FY11, NCB-Prepared achieved their overarching objective to build a proof of concept for the state of North Carolina using a scalable cloud-computing platform that provides access to data and data visualization using a rules-based technology to support data quality and security. The project created new data discovery and integration methodologies that helped address long-standing challenges in the quality and completeness of data records and yielded improved sensitivity and specificity of existing analytical tools for health threat detection. These discoveries and methodologies will be evaluated for operational adoption by NBIC and incorporated as appropriate to improve the NBIC.

In FY12 and FY 13, NCB-Prepared will develop an operational system that canvases three states, including North Carolina, South Carolina and West Virginia, to provide alerts and warnings at the state level but scalable to provide a national biosurveillance picture. This regional collaboration will link directly to NBIC to improve information sharing with state and local stakeholders. It will provide NBIC a better understanding for the utility of state information and the value NBIC can provide to the states.

In FY13, NCB-Prepared will continue to incorporate additional states into its states and national biosurveillance data sets for the trusted third party network. NCB-Prepared will further its network and establish a means for sustainability outside of the federal government. Should metrics for success be met by FY14, NCB-Prepared data and analysis will be regularly shared and operationally integrated into NBIC.

Activity 2.2.2. NBIC Ingest Information Technology Tools

In FY12, NBIC is assessing potential IT capabilities to enhance current operations of the NBIS. Several pilot projects touch on "information sharing and integration" and "collaboration", however, most of these pilots remain in the requirements definition phase. As part of the assessment, NBIC has released a request for information (RFI) to industry to identify potential capabilities. NBIC is in the process of reviewing the industry white papers that were submitted to determine any possible further action in FY13.

Activity 2.2.3. Function-based Pilot Program: Social Media

Social networking is an open, inclusive bridge encouraging the exchange of real time information around the world that is routinely postulated as having biosurveillance value. The capability has undergone small scale investigations in academia, but has not been thoroughly tested in a national operations environment. Thus, one of the pilot programs that OHA will explore from FY12 through the end of FY13 is to scientifically evaluate the value of social media in biosurveillance. This pilot's goals are to determine the early warning and event characterization value of social media. The program will test and evaluate specific analytical tools and compare performance to known social media analysis providers such as Google Flu.

OHA will examine if social media can augment existing biosurveillance detection and analysis capabilities of the government through either earlier advance warning or better characterization of an ongoing event. This effort will examine initiatives undertaken by other NBIS partners and leverage them where possible.

Activity 2.2.4. Private Sector Absenteeism

Private companies with a large number of employees are potential early indicators of biological events. Their sampling size when spread over large parts of the United States could serve as a barometer pointing to early detection of biological events of national concern. Normally, unstructured data on sickness is gathered in a structured form when these large companies analyze their absenteeism rates. A number of biosurveillance systems are available or under development, including information regarding emergency service use, consumer complaints, over-the-counter medication sales, employee absenteeism, and use of social media.

In FY13 through FY14, the NBIC will explore how it can partner with private industry to test the trigger mechanism that a large representative group of employees provides. Absenteeism trends could reinforce biosurveillance goals of ever earlier detection and increased situational awareness to reduce the intensity and duration of a biological event. In conjunction with DHS Infrastructure Protection's Protected Critical Infrastructure Information program, the NBIC will partner with the private sector in this promising initiative.

In addition, in FY12 through FY13, NBIC will continue work with DHS Chief Human Capital Officer to regularly receive de-identified DHS absenteeism data. As a large employer with over 250,000 employees, trend data from DHS may provide a sample size large enough provide surveillance benefits and to encourage NBIS partners to analyze similar data within their own departments and agencies.

Strategic Objective 2.3

Incorporate information technology systems that use the best available statistical and other analytical tools to identify, characterize, localize, and track biological events of national concern in as close to real time as is feasible.

Activity 2.3.1. FDA Food Safety Modernization Act Implementation

The Food Safety Modernization Act states, "The [HHS] Secretary, acting through the Director of the Centers for Disease Control and Prevention [CDC], shall enhance foodborne illness surveillance systems to improve the collection, analysis, reporting, and usefulness of data on foodborne illnesses." The list of ways this mandate should be met includes "integrating foodborne illness surveillance systems and data with other biosurveillance and public health situational awareness capabilities at the federal, state, and local levels, including by sharing foodborne illness surveillance data with the National Biosurveillance Integration Center.[26]"

1. The legislation specifically uses the word "data" versus "information," suggesting the intent is to move beyond summary reports and a possible need for a robust information technology sharing interface. This requires a long-term OHA commitment to data integration with our partners.
2. At this time, HHS/CDC and NBIC are exploring how to implement the legislation consistent with the CDC and NBIC information sharing focus.

Activity 2.3.2. Current Information Technology-based Biosurveillance Capabilities

The BCON and the BCOP are the two primary Information Technology tools used by the NBIC analysts to perform daily biosurveillance.

BCON initiatives include:

- In FY12, NBIC has awarded a contract to externally review the utility of BCON. Within five months of award, a decision will be presented to the NBIC for continued use of the BCON system as-is, a transition plan for a replacement ingest tool, or migration of BCON management to another organization such as DHS OCIO.

BCOP initiatives include:

- Expansion of the BCOP user interface fixes: back navigation, single log-in, and certificates.
- Working with other OHA partners, BioWatch and the Health Security Intelligence Enterprise, to have their portals route users directly to BCOP.
- Leverage the input from the Association of State and Territorial Health Officials to provide feedback and updated requirements on the advancement of the BCOP system.
- Investigate other potential future hosts for the BCOP to include the NOC COP

These enhancements are in response to customer inputs and will take place during FY12 and FY13. The NBIC will continue to work within NBIS partner current IT capabilities and seek opportunities to leverage information sharing with them.

Activity 2.3.3. National Poison Data System

The NBIC will work to include the Association of American Poison Control Center (AAPCC) personnel and information in the NBIS analysis process. While CDC currently collaborates with the AAPCC, poison control data has not previously been fully operationalized. NBIC and CDC will collaborate to enhance operationalization, sharing AAPCC-generated alerts with the interagency. NBIC will use real time AAPCC data to share information on known or suspected biological agent, toxin, and chemical exposures and effects.

Strategic Goal 3

Enhance federal government ability to disseminate alerts and other information to NBIS partner agencies and to agencies of state, local, and tribal governments.

Congress charges the NBIC to disseminate biosurveillance information. The NBIC enhances shared situational awareness and provides decision making support through user-defined reporting. This reporting is shaped by stakeholders and built from the collaboration, information integration, and analysis from across the NBIS partners. As a core discipline, effective information dissemination to the appropriate people in the appropriate user-defined format is critical in accomplishing this goal.

Strategic Objective 3.1

Strengthen and mature the method of real time communication with the NOC and provide 24 hour support to the NOC.

Activity 3.1.1. DHS National Operations Center Common Operating Picture

In FY12, NBIC and OCIO are working to nest biosurveillance information within the NOC COP so that this information is available to the federal interagency as well as SLTT entities. NBIC and OCIO are defining the requirements through participation on the NOC COP integrated product team. Concurrently migrating DHS biosurveillance data/information from operational components to the NOC COP will provide more defined roles and responsibilities between the NOC and NBIC. This effort will enhance the ability to conduct NBIC Protocol Activations and clarify the relationship between NBIC and the NOC to NBIS member agencies.

As a first step, in order to clarify the distinct roles of OHA as a member of the NBIS and OHA as a representative of the Department's Chief Medical Officer, there will be two representatives to the NOC CAT to properly fill the duties to each organization. An NBIS representative will be nominated by the NBIC to serve on the CAT specifically for coordinating NOC requirements with executing the biosurveillance mission. NBIC will continue to monitor event tempo among the NBIS partners and communicate regularly through the CAT.

Activity 3.1.2. FEMA Emergency Notification System

The NBIC implemented use of the FEMA Emergency Notification System for NBIS Protocol activations during FY12. This upgrade allows for notification of a scheduled teleconference to all participants within several minutes via phone and email.

Strategic Objective 3.2

Implement information sharing in consultation with the Office of the Director of National Intelligence, DHS Under Secretary for Intelligence & Analysis (I&A), and other U.S. government entities, as appropriate.

Activity 3.2.1. Security Clearances and Facility Clearances

From FY12 through the end of FY13, as part of a wider workforce analysis, OHA will evaluate the proportion of NBIC staff with high-level top secret/sensitive compartmented information clearances and sensitive compartmented information facility access to ensure that the NBIC effectively meets the requirements in P.L. 110-53 regarding coordination with the NOC and the broader intelligence community.

Activity 3.2.2. Intelligence Community Outreach Strategy

P.L. 110-53 directs that the NBIC conduct notifications, assessments, and information sharing "in consultation with the Director of National Intelligence, the Under Secretary for Intelligence and Analysis, and other offices or agencies of the federal government, as appropriate." NBIC continues to improve its coordination with the broader intelligence community to include coordination with the National Center for Medical Intelligence, to whom OHA has assigned a liaison.

NBIC needs to combine the access of appropriate security clearances for its analysts with the benefit that comes from being physically co-located with an intelligence agency. The Congressional charge to implement information sharing in consultation with the Office of the Director of National Intelligence can be accomplished by leveraging the Department's resident intelligence Component.

- In FY12, NBIC will establish a formal relationship with DHS I&A to receive, be informed of, and analyze classified products. Leveraging the existing relationship between OHA's State and Local Initiatives office and DHS I&A, OHA will draft a memorandum of understanding (MOU) between OHA and I&A for sharing of classified biosurveillance products.

Strategic Goal 4

Mature and Strengthen NBIC into a World-class Biosurveillance Analysis and Integration Organization.

This strategic plan forms the first framework for a review of the alignment of NBIC resources with core mission activities as expressed in the strategic goals and objectives. Strategic planning will help enhance the NBIC's collaboration, information sharing and integration, analysis, and user-defined reporting capabilities. The NBIC's initial development over the past four years with the collaborative effort of NBIS partners and the broader biosurveillance community over the past year inform this strategic plan and the resource requirements.

The NBIC will produce an annual update to the five-year plan in the fall of each year to accompany its budget submission. This is an emerging strategy that requires periodic review, in which NBIS partners will be invited to participate.

Strategic Objective 4.1

Recruit, develop, and retain a collaborative, talented, multi-disciplinary analytic staff with the necessary expertise to develop and operate the NBIC.

Activity 4.1.1. Recruit, Develop, and Retain a Cadre of DHS Biosurveillance Professionals to Operate the NBIC

Public Law 110-53 states: "The Directing Officer of the NBIC shall hire individuals with the necessary expertise to develop and operate the NBIC" and directs the NBIC to evaluate the analytical capability of NBIC on an ongoing basis. Successful analysis of large, disparate sources of data and information to produce early warning and shared situational awareness regarding biological events requires a diverse, multidisciplinary staff trained to produce and integrate relevant and timely analysis for decision makers. As the budget and staffing allows, NBIC will recruit and retain a highly skilled staff through processes which include but are not limited to standard hiring processes, the Public Health Service, and fellowship programs such as the Presidential Management Fellows.

Though NBIC analysts have gained immeasurable institutional knowledge and refined their analytical capabilities of biosurveillance information during their tenure, this 2007 assessment requires revision. In order to address the expertise needed for the entirety of the biosphere, biosurveillance integration and operations, the NBIC must have the right number of the right kinds of analysts to include all necessary areas of expertise.

Strategic Objective 4.2

To augment the expertise of NBIC biosurveillance professionals in Strategic Objective 4.1, recruit technical expertise in human, animal, plant, food, and environmental information analysis and interpretation through interagency agreements and other vehicles.

Biosurveillance integration occurs within the analysis and production section of the NBIC. The NBIC's subject matter experts work with NBIS liaison officers who reach back using the vast analytic capability of their departments. Robust collaboration across the federal, SLTT, and private domains occurs at the intersection where NBIC analysts, NBIS Liaison Officers, real time communications with the NOC, and robust collaboration with DHS I&A and broader intelligence communities converge.

Activity 4.2.1. Member Agency Memorandum of Understanding

NBIC seeks to complete MOUs with all NBIS partners by the end of FY13. The level of NBIS participation of partners varies depending on whether a partner is a net consumer or producer of biosurveillance information. Likewise, each MOU reflect the diverse capabilities and levels of biosurveillance effort of the NBIS partners.

Activity 4.2.2. NBIC Interagency Agreements (IAAs)

Congress directs Member Agencies to "provide personnel to the NBIC under an interagency personnel agreement and consider the qualifications of such personnel necessary to provide human, animal, and environmental data analysis and interpretation support to the NBIC." The NBIC is authorized to reimburse any department or agency providing personnel and will continue to seek liaison officer representation from all federal NBIS partners. Not all NBIS partners perform biosurveillance at the same scope, or in the same way. Therefore, the need for an IAA will vary as well as the level of participation under IAAs.

The NBIC leverages LNOs who enhance collaboration and integration with NBIS partners. The LNO presence is defined by each partner. Placement can vary from full-time presence at the NBIC to part-time or virtual. Virtual LNOs could provide regular agency points of contact while maintaining presence at the LNO's home agency. On site, the NBIC has one LNO from

USDA FSIS and has continued to increase federal agency engagement through OHA liaison officer positions. The CDC has provided an LNO to OHA since the start of FY12. In addition, DHS S&T has provided an LNO to the Armed Forces Health Surveillance Center since the start of FY12. The NBIC has been able to leverage this position to increase its engagement with the Department of Defense. Furthermore, OHA has been providing an LNO to the National Center for Medical Intelligence since the start of FY12. An LNO from the Department of Veteran Affairs is expected to join the NBIC in 2012.

- Given the nature of NBIC's mission, Public Health Service officers are anticipated to be an essential component of the NBIC team, providing expertise in medicine and public health.
- In FY12, the NBIC will seek an LNO from the National Wildlife Health Center (NWHC). The NWHC is part of the U.S. Geological Survey within the Department of the Interior. The mission of the NWHC is to provide information, technical assistance, and research associated with global wildlife health issues. Among other activities, the NWHC is engaged in monitoring and assessing the impact of disease on wildlife, as well as defining ecological relationships affecting disease occurrence. The NBIC will seek to have an on-site LNO in place in FY13.

Strategic Objective 4.3

Support the growth and development of a cadre of DHS biosurveillance professionals through training opportunities.

Activity 4.3.1. Biosurveillance Workforce of the Future

This objective draws directly from the National Biosurveillance Strategy for Human Health priority area of the biosurveillance workforce of the future. One of the challenges in developing this workforce is getting access to specialists. "Professionals performing biosurveillance need access to specialists such as statisticians, epidemiologic and mathematical modelers, information and decision scientists, informaticians, natural language processing experts, analytic data management programmers, knowledge managers, and disease and GIS mapping experts."[27] The NBIC will seek continuing professional development opportunities for its analysts and other biosurveillance professionals in the broader community beginning in FY13.

Activity 4.3.2. Operations-to-Operations Exchange

The NBIC will provide professional development opportunities to its analysts to advance awareness of and cooperation within the interagency biosurveillance community. The analysts will be detailed to federal NBIS partner agencies and other organizations for up to two-week exchanges biannually. The agency targeted will reflect the subject matter expertise of each analyst. This will permit the NBIC's analysts to better understand the mission of NBIS partners, learn the processes and challenges of these agencies, and to develop professional contacts to enhance future collaboration. Other exchanges could include laboratories or Centers of Excellence. Continuing exchanges outside staff areas of expertise will continue to provide broadening of biosurveillance experience.

CONCLUSION

Effective management of risks from biological threats and hazards depends on early warning and shared situational awareness, so that risk management decisions surrounding response and recovery are well-informed. To that end, the federal government performs biosurveillance through several domains: human, animal, plant, food, and environmental health. The federal government has the duty to ensure that information from across these domains is analyzed, shared, and used in ways that save lives, ensure civil order and preserve government, mitigate socioeconomic impacts, and reduce the likelihood of reoccurring events. Within that duty, the NBIC has a key responsibility to integrate the nation's biosurveillance information. Every day the NBIC reaches back through federal partners and SLTT stakeholders as well as the private sector to enhance the federal government's capability to integrate and share biosurveillance information in support of decision makers. There is still much to be learned from combining these different information sources.

This Strategic Plan groups the NBIC biosurveillance effort into four core disciplines which include: 1) Collaboration, in which governance improvements and new communication processes and policies will be pursued; 2) Information integration and sharing, in which appropriate IT systems, business rules, and partner data management/ownership verification will be a priority, 3) Analysis, which requires multidisciplinary, cross-cutting, and in-depth analytic support to provide timely and relevant information to support decisions; and 4) User-defined reporting, recognizing that all aspects of the NBIC's analysis and products must be tailored and customer-focused.

Having a strong, state-of-the-art NBIC will support these efforts on behalf of the community, and this Strategic Plan articulates clear strategic goals, objectives, and activities essential to achieving its mission. Through the NBIC, and working together with our partners and stakeholders, we will advance the safety, security, and resilience of the nation through leadership in biosurveillance integration.

ANNEX A: AUTHORITIES

1. Implementing Recommendations of the 9/11 Commission Act of 2007, Public Law 110-53, 121 Stat. 266 (2007), codified in part at 6 USC §195b, "National Biosurveillance Integration Center"
2. FDA Food Safety Modernization Act of 2011, Public Law 111-353, 124 Stat. 388, sec. 205, codified in 21 U.S.C. 2224 (2011).
3. Homeland Security Presidential Directive 9 – Establishes a national policy to defend the agriculture and food system against terrorist attacks, major disasters, and other emergencies.
4. Homeland Security Presidential Directive 10 – Provides a comprehensive framework for our nation's biodefense.
5. Homeland Security Presidential Directive 21 – Establishes a national strategy that will enable a level of public health and medical preparedness sufficient to address a range of possible disasters.

ANNEX B: ACRONYMS

AAPCC	Association of American Poison Control Center
BCON	Biosurveillance Common Operating Network
BCOP	Biosurveillance Common Operating Picture
BIWAC	Biological Indicators and Warnings Advisory Committee
CAT	Crisis Action Team
CDC	Centers for Disease Control and Prevention
CIR	Critical Information Requirements
CONOPS	Concept of Operations

COP	Common Operating Picture
DHS	Department of Homeland Security
FAVD	Food, Agriculture, and Veterinary Defense
FDA	Food and Drug Administration
FSIS	Food Safety and Inspection Service
GAO	Government Accountability Office
HHS	Health and Human Services
HSIN	Homeland Security Information Network
HSPD	Homeland Security Presidential Directives
I&A	Intelligence and Analysis
IAA	Interagency Agreement
IHR	International Health Regulations
ISA	Information Sharing Agreements
IT	Information Technology
LNO	Liaison Officer
MOU	Memorandum of Understanding
NBIC	National Biosurveillance Integration Center
NBIS	National Biosurveillance Integration System
NCB-Prepared	National Collaborative for Bio-Preparedness
NCFPD	National Center for Food Protection and Defense Center of Excellence
NIOC	NBIS Interagency Oversight Council
NIWG	NBIS Interagency Working Group
NOC	National Operations Center
NSS	National Security Staff
NWHC	National Wildlife Health Center
OCIO	Office of the Chief Information Officer
OHA	Office of Health Affairs
PHEIC	Public Health Emergency of International Concern
PPD	Presidential Policy Directive
RFI	Requests for Information
RSS	Really Simple Syndication
SLTT	State, local, territorial, tribal
SME	Subject Matter Expert
USDA	U.S. Department of Agriculture
WHO	World Health Organization

End Notes

[1] The term "biological event of national concern is defined in Public Law 110-53: to mean—"(A) an act of terrorism involving a biological agent or toxin; or "(B) a naturally occurring outbreak of an infectious disease that may result in a national epidemic." For the purposes of NBIC, biological spans a variety of domains to include the health of humans, animals, and plants, as well as the safety and security of food and the environment.

[2] In the context of this document, shared situational awareness is established through the integration and sharing of biosurveillance information and part of the larger situational awareness established by the National Operations Center Common Operating Picture.

[3] "Events" includes naturally-occurring, accidental, or deliberate biological events such as emerging infectious disease or bioterrorism.

[4] Core Disciplines have been formulated based on numerous Government Accountability Office reports on biosurveillance and through internal review and discussion with key stakeholders.

[5] The White House, "Biodefense for the 21st Century," Homeland Security Presidential Directive 10, April 28, 2004. Accessed online at http://www.fas.org/irp/offdocs/nspd/hspd-10.html.

[6] Public Law 110-53: The term 'biological event of national concern' means—''(A) an act of terrorism involving a biological agent or toxin; or ''(B) a naturally occurring outbreak of an infectious disease that may result in a national epidemic."

[7] Public Law 111-353, section 205(b)(1).

[8] PPD-8 defines five preparedness mission areas—Prevention, Protection, Mitigation, Response, and Recovery. Information regarding the deliverables of PPD-8 are located online at http://www.fema.gov/prepared/ppd8.shtm.

[9] The White House, *National Strategy for Biosurveillance*, July 2012. Accessed online at http://www.whitehouse.gov/sites/default/files/National_Strategy_for_Biosurveillance_July_2012.pdf.

[10] "Biosphere data" can be divided into information about human, animal, and agricultural populations, and biosurveillance thus consists of health surveillance on each of these populations. Cited from Ronald D. Fricker, "Biosurveillance: Detecting, Tracking, and Mitigating the Effects of Natural Disease and Bioterrorism," Naval Post Graduate School (2010): 2.

[11] The White House, "Public Health and Medical Preparedness," Homeland Security Presidential Directive 21, October 18, 2007. Accessed online at http://www.fas.org/irp/offdocs/nspd/hspd-21.htm.

[12] Mica Endsley, Toward a theory of situation awareness in dynamic systems (Human Factors, 1995b), 32-64.

[13] Concept established through integration of two theories: Endsley, M. R. Designing for Situation Awareness: An Approach to User-Centered Design (CRC Press, 2003) and Nofi, Albert A. Defining and Measuring Shared Situational Awareness (Center for Naval Analyses Corporation, 2000).

[14] Core Disciplines have been formulated based on numerous Government Accountability Office reports on biosurveillance and through internal review and discussion with key stakeholders.

[15] Collaboration as a Core Disciple of Integrated Biosurveillance is in alignment with the *Planning* Core Capability of the PPD-8 National Preparedness Goal.

[16] Recommendation identified in the Government Accountability Office, *Report on Biosurveillance: Developing a Collaboration Strategy is Essential to Fostering Interagency Data and Resource Sharing,* GAO 10-171(Washington, DC: GAO, 2009).

[17] Information Integration and Sharing as a Core Disciple of Integrated Biosurveillance is in alignment with the *Public Information and Warning* Core Capability of the PPD-8 National Preparedness Goal.

[18] Information regarding this activity as led by the Centers for Disease Control and Prevention is highlighted in the GAO-10-645: *Report on Biosurveillance: Efforts to Develop a National Biosurveillance Capability Need a National Strategy and a Designated Leader'* (Washington, DC: GAO 10-645, 2010).

[19] Analysis and User-Defined Reporting as Core Disciples of Integrated Biosurveillance is in alignment with the *Operational Coordination* Core Capability of the PPD-8 National Preparedness Goal.

[20] According to the Delegation to the Assistant Secretary from the DHS Secretary July 24, 2008, the authority includes but is not limited to (1) leading DHS' biodefense activities, to include oversight and management for implementation of HSPD-10; (2) managing DHS' operational biodefense programs.

[21] U.S. Department of Homeland Security. *Quadrennial Homeland Security Review Report: A Strategic Framework for a Secure Homeland.* Page 2. February 2010.

[22] U.S. Department of Homeland Security. *DHS Risk Lexicon.* September 2010.

[23] OHA recognizes the contributions the Biological Indications and Warning Analytic Community (BIWAC) has made and continues to make and will incorporate lessons learned as appropriate.

[24] Recommendation identified in the Government Accountability Office, *Report on Biosurveillance: Developing a Collaboration Strategy is Essential to Fostering Interagency Data and Resource Sharing,* GAO 10-171(Washington, DC: GAO, 2009).

[25] The addition of a co-chair will not alter or impede the OHA Assistant Secretary's or NBIC's statutory authorities outlined in the 6 U.S.C. § 321e and 6 U.S.C. § 195b.

[26] Public Law 111-353, section 205(b)(1).

[27] U.S. Department of Health and Human Services. *National Biosurveillance Strategy for Human Health.* February 2010.

INDEX

#

A

B

C

D

E

S

T

U

V

W